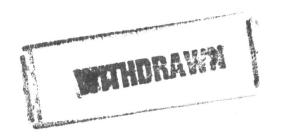

UTERINE
FIBROIDS

A Johns Hopkins Press Health Book

UTERINE FIBROIDS

The Complete Guide

Elizabeth A. Stewart, M.D.

THE JOHNS HOPKINS UNIVERSITY PRESS
Baltimore

Note to the Reader

This book is not meant to substitute for the medical care of women with fibroid tumors, and treatment should not be based solely on its contents. Instead, treatment must be developed in a dialogue between the individual and her physician. This book has been written to help with that dialogue.

Drug dosage: The author and publisher have made reasonable efforts to determine that the selection and dosage of drugs discussed in this text conform to the practices of the general medical community. The medications described do not necessarily have specific approval by the U.S. Food and Drug Administration for use in the diseases and dosages for which they are recommended. In view of ongoing research, changes in governmental regulations, and the constant flow of information relating to drug therapy and drug reactions, the reader is urged to check the package insert of each drug for any change in indications and dosage and for warnings and precautions. This is particularly important when the recommended agent is a new and/or infrequently used drug.

© 2007 Elizabeth A. Stewart
All rights reserved. Published 2007
Printed in the United States of America on acid-free paper
9 8 7 6 5 4 3 2 1

The Johns Hopkins University Press
2715 North Charles Street
Baltimore, Maryland 21218-4363
www.press.jhu.edu

Library of Congress Cataloging-in-Publication Data
Stewart, Elizabeth A.
    Uterine fibroids: the complete guide / Elizabeth A. Stewart.
      p. cm.
    Includes bibliographical references and index.
    ISBN-13: 978-0-8018-8700-0 (hardcover : alk. paper)
    ISBN-13: 978-0-8018-8701-7 (pbk. : alk. paper)
    ISBN-10: 0-8018-8700-3 (hardcover : alk. paper)
    ISBN-10: 0-8018-8701-1 (pbk.: alk. paper)
    1. Uterine Fibroids. 1. Title.
    RC280.U8S75 2007
    616.99'366—dc22   2006103536

A catalog record for this book is available from the British Library.

Special discounts are available for bulk purchases of this book. For more information, please contact Special Sales at 410-516-6936 or specialsales@press.jhu.edu.

All illustrations and photographic overlays by Jacqueline Schaffer

To Bill and Paul

*Both ahead of their time in their support of women and
the unique issues women face.*

Contents

Part III. Medical Treatment

Part IV. Other Factors, Other Conditions

Introduction

Fibroids (or, in medical parlance, leiomyomas, myomas, or leiomyomata) are basically knots of smooth muscle in the uterine wall. As Natalie Angier noted in her wonderful book titled *Woman: An Intimate Geography*, "Fibroids are as common as freckles and deserve their common name."[1] They are found to be present in at least 25 percent of all women, and they would be found in over 80 percent of all women if one looked carefully enough. Fibroids are the leading reason for a hysterectomy, accounting for more hysterectomies than all kinds of gynecologic cancers put together. Despite this high prevalence, we know much less about them than we do about the smooth muscle cells in the lungs that contribute to asthma or the smooth muscle cells in the heart or blood vessels involved in coronary artery disease. Fibroids clearly deserve more scientific investigation. They have been the focus of my work as a scientist and a practicing gynecologist.

Why write a book about fibroids? For me, there are many personal reasons.

First, the field is changing rapidly. Making decisions about treatment options was easy when hysterectomy was the one-size-fits-all treatment. But as a headline from a news article a few years ago succinctly stated, "Diagnosing fibroids is simple. Deciding what to do is hard."[2] Today, in making a decision about treatment, many factors come into play: how many fibroids are present, their size and location, what symptoms I am having, my plans for pregnancy in the future, to name a few.

Second, women are increasingly sophisticated in their approach to making decisions for themselves and their loved ones. The Internet has been a great boon to this process. My patients now come in with a sophisticated understanding of the disease process and the appropriate treatment options. Many of them have figured out the best treatment for their particular situation, and their specific questions may be more enlightened than the ones asked by medical students rotating through my office. The problem is that Web sites often don't disclose their biases. And they are often tailored to recommend one specific therapy—in effect saying, "I do procedure X for fibroids, and therefore everyone should have procedure X."

Being self-educated in advance of a consultation with a physician is becoming increasingly critical because the time allotted to appointments becomes shorter with each passing year due to the pressures of the economics of health care. Even over the course of my twenty-year career in gynecology I find that I am always trying to convey more information in a shorter time. I developed a variety of handouts on specific topics to try to handle this pressure, and those handouts were the seeds from which this book has grown. My travels have convinced me that, unfortunately, less than optimum doctor-patient communication will continue. In most other countries, doctors can't take time to talk with patients. Their specialized skills are deployed in the most cost-effective way to perform physical exams and do procedures. In some ways, health care is like the manufacturing of toothpaste, but the art of medicine is something that is disappearing with increasing focus on productivity.

Finally, nothing beats personal experience to promote both understanding and empathy. When a physician has been "the patient," the interaction becomes a partnership. Experiences with illness and the health care system teach you things you will never learn in medical school or practice. Many of the lessons I have learned about pain management and postoperative recovery I learned trying to deal with one of my seven surgeries. (See the Appendix for some hints about recovering from surgery.)

My hope is that many of the lessons I have learned will help other women move forward to health and that women in my daughter's generation will have better options.

PART I

About Fibroids

CHAPTER 1

Who Gets Fibroids, and What Are the Symptoms?

The two most common symptoms associated with fibroids are heavy menstrual periods (termed *menorrhagia*) and pelvic pressure or discomfort. (There is a movement away from using these older words, such as menorrhagia, to make the terminology more understandable.) Menorrhagia involves periods that are either long or heavy or both. Typical menstrual periods last 4 to 5 days, so, generally, any woman who has 7 or more days of menstrual bleeding is considered to have menorrhagia. Some women have relatively short periods (in the range of 3 to 4 days), but their periods are excessively heavy.

There is no good classification system for the heaviness of periods. When I was a student, one of the senior doctors said that whenever he got a call from a patient complaining of heavy bleeding, he would ask whether the bleeding was so heavy that blood would fill up her shoes if she were standing without a pad. If she replied that it was, he would ask her to come in immediately. Although an exchange like this would be considered patronizing today, it does illustrate the difficulty of describing excessive bleeding. There are other ways to get an assessment of heavy menstrual bleeding, but there are no good studies looking at the reliability of these measures.

The following commonly occur in women with fibroids and heavy menstrual bleeding:

- Needing to change a pad or a tampon more frequently than every two hours.

- Needing to use double sanitary protection (a pad and a tampon, or two pads or two tampons) frequently.
- Wearing adult diapers for menstrual control.
- *Flooding* is the common term for loss of control of menstrual flow. Even with the maximal use of pads and/or tampons, when flooding occurs, women may still have menstrual accidents that stain their clothes.
- With heavy flow, women also typically get up at night to change sanitary protection or frequently soil their bedclothes.
- Many women deal with the heavy menstrual flow by changing their work or social schedule. Any change in your schedule because of your menstrual period is likely to mean that you have significant menstrual flow.

It is also important to check whether a woman with fibroids has anemia (a low red blood cell count). Several different tests can be ordered, including a hematocrit, a hemoglobin, or a complete blood count (CBC). An old notion stipulates that if a woman is not anemic, she cannot have significant menstrual bleeding. But many women are able to maintain normal blood counts with iron, vitamins, and diet despite substantial blood loss. Conversely, some women don't feel that they are having heavy bleeding, but they develop significant anemia from their periods.

The second common symptom associated with fibroids is pelvic pressure or discomfort. This typically is not sharp or disabling pain but rather discomfort based on the size of the uterus and the pressure the uterus causes on adjacent organs as illustrated in figure 1.1. It is similar to the discomfort pregnant women have because fibroids enlarge the uterus to sizes commonly seen in pregnancy. Just like pregnant women, women with fibroids can have urinary frequency, difficulty with bowel movements or constipation, difficulty emptying their bladder completely, back pain, abdominal distention, sciatica (pain radiating from the buttocks down the back of the leg), and bloating. The fibroids can become quite large before the woman recognizes these problems. The slow development of the fibroids over time probably accounts for this delay in perception. Pregnant women at 5 months know that their symptoms are different from before they were pregnant; however, a woman with a 5-month-sized fibroid uterus may have had it steadily grow over 5 to 10 years, and therefore she mistakenly attributes the changes to other processes, such as aging.

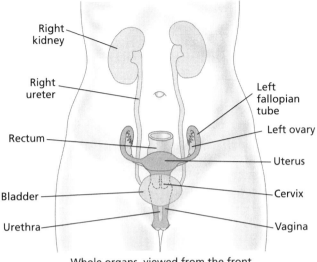

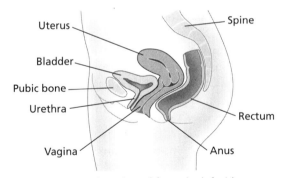

Figure 1.1. The uterus is in the pelvis and thus is normally not felt by pushing on the abdomen. This is why a pelvic exam is performed as a part of gynecologic care. The bladder is in front of the uterus and rests on the lower part of the uterus and upper cervix. The bowel (rectum) is behind the uterus. When the body is viewed in cross section, the bladder is in front of the uterus, which in turn is in front of the rectum. Each of these important pelvic structures also leads to an opening on the perineum: the bladder terminates in the urethra, the uterus in the vagina, and the rectum in the anus. When looking at the perineum, as is done when a woman has a pelvic exam and is lying on her back, these openings go from top to bottom, so that the urethra is most superior, the vagina is below that, and the anus is the bottommost opening. The ureters carry urine from the kidneys (located in the back above the belly button, termed the *flank*) to the bladder and thus pass to either side of the uterus.

Sudden or severe pain can occasionally occur with fibroids. These symptoms typically occur under two circumstances. The first is when the fibroid grows faster than its blood supply and the center of the fibroid dies or degenerates. This can happen to any type of fibroid. The second circumstance for acute pain occurs with a pedunculated fibroid (a fibroid on a stalk). If the fibroid twists on its stalk, it can cut off blood supply and cause sudden pain. However, given the perception that sharp, severe pain is uncommon with fibroids, before concluding that fibroids are a source of acute pain, other causes should be investigated, including an ovarian cyst or endometriosis. Some information coming from studies of women undergoing uterine artery embolization as a treatment for fibroids suggests that pain with fibroids may be more common than previously thought.

Reproductive dysfunction, including infertility, miscarriage, and pregnancy complications, can also be associated with fibroids. However, most women with fibroids get pregnant without difficulty and have uncomplicated pregnancies and deliveries. Again, before attributing reproductive difficulties to a fibroid, a thorough investigation of the woman and her partner should take place to exclude other, more common causes. Difficulty getting pregnant (infertility) or problems with early miscarriages are most commonly seen with fibroids that distort the endometrial cavity (submucosal fibroids).[1,2] Luckily, these fibroids are the ones that are most easily treated in a minimally invasive fashion with a hysteroscope.

Fibroids can sometimes cause problems during pregnancy (this subject is discussed in detail in Chapter 18). These complications of pregnancy are more likely with larger fibroids and with fibroids that are located directly beneath the placenta. The pregnancy complications that have been associated with fibroids include the following:

- Bleeding in the first trimester
- Increased risk of cesarean section
- Increased risk of preterm labor
- Increased risk of placental abruption

We don't precisely know why the size of the fibroid and the location of the placenta in relation to the fibroid are critical to pregnancy complications. I like to use the analogy of planting a tree in soil that has a large rock beneath it. While initially it may be fine, as the roots get established, the tree will not flourish. The placenta grows into the uterine wall, and if it has a large mass at its base, its growth may be impeded, a situation similar to what happens with the tree.

A second issue related to pregnancy complications may be that (as discussed in Chapter 2) the microscopic composition of the endometrium (lining of the uterus) and the molecules produced in the endometrium of women with uterine fibroids may be abnormal. The process of a pregnancy implanting in the uterus involves a "molecular dialogue" between the embryo and the endometrium. The embryo looks for and responds to specific signals from the uterus. Either the fibroid may misdirect the embryo to a less favorable place for implantation, or the endometrium may be lacking in a specific component required for implantation or pregnancy success.

A final problem with fibroids (not related to pregnancy) is that, rarely, fibroids can become so large that they place pressure on the ureters, which carry urine from the kidneys to the bladder. Sometimes if this pressure is severe and there is damage to the kidneys (moderate or severe hydronephrosis), even fibroids that are not causing symptoms need to be removed.

How Common Are Uterine Fibroids?

Studies show that up to 80 percent of women have fibroids in their uterus.[3]* This figure comes from microscopic study of uteruses (also termed uteri) removed at the time of surgery and uteruses removed from women who died of nongynecologic causes. Thus, it is likely that most, if not all, women have some microscopic fibroids in their uterus.

The percentage of women with clinically significant uterine fibroids (ones large enough to be felt on pelvic exams or visualized on ultrasound) is commonly reported to be approximately 25 percent. Calculating 25 percent of women between the ages of 19 and 64 from recent census figures for the U.S. population would mean that 23 million women might be estimated to have fibroids. However, this percentage varies with how thoroughly women are evaluated to

---

*Note: In this book, when I say "Studies show" or "Studies suggest" or "There is some evidence," I am referring to the results of scientific studies. When I am describing my own clinical practice, or my own impressions based on my practice, I indicate that fact, as well.

find fibroids. Thus, studies that report only fibroids felt on pelvic exam will underestimate fibroids compared with studies that use ultrasound. It is clear, however, that black women have an increased risk of having fibroids (termed *prevalence*).[4] They also appear to develop fibroids at three times the rate of Caucasian women (termed *incidence*).[4]

There is some evidence that black women with fibroids also develop more severe disease and do so at an earlier age.[5] A study has estimated that up to 80 percent of African American women in the United States will develop ultrasound-detectable fibroids.[6] Although large-scale studies have not been conducted in Africa, it appears that African women have a similar risk of fibroids. The studies that have been done to date also suggest that this increased prevalence and incidence are not due to other confounding factors (factors that would vary between African American and Caucasian women and would account for this difference, such as age at first pregnancy, height, and weight).[4]

Factors That Can Influence a Woman's Chance of Developing Uterine Fibroids

Race can affect your risk. As discussed in the previous section, being African American appears to lead to an increase in risk of fibroids. Hispanic and Asian women appear to have the same risk as Caucasian women. However, the number of Hispanic and Asian women in the studies done to date has been small.[7] It is also not clear whether there is a difference between women in Africa and African American women in terms of fibroid risk. Most of the studies to date have been done in the United States or Europe, but it does appear that women in Africa also have significant problems with fibroids.

Having *close relatives with fibroids* appears to increase risk. This factor is called *familial clustering,* and it suggests that there may be a genetic reason for developing fibroids.[8,9]

Delivering a baby leads to a decreased risk of uterine fibroids.[10–12] Having delivered a baby is termed *parity.* We do not understand why pregnancy decreases the risk of fibroid formation, but some scientists cite the remodeling of the uterus that takes place following pregnancy as possibly clearing newly formed fibroids.[13]

Some studies suggest that taking *oral contraceptive pills* may decrease the risk of fibroid formation.[10,14,15] Many textbooks continue to say that women with fibroids should not take birth control pills because of the concern that the fibroids might grow rapidly. Although this can happen, many fibroids do not grow over time. The difference in findings is likely explained by the fact that, once established, the fibroids can respond to the hormones in the pills; on the other hand, the steady state of hormones in the pill may prevent cells from forming fibroids or fibroids from starting the growth process. The timing of beginning the birth control pill may be critical. In the large Nurses' Health Study most women on pills had a decreased risk of fibroids, but women starting pills between the ages of 13 and 16 actually had an increased risk.[7, 15]

Smoking also decreases the risk of fibroids, possibly because of differences in estrogen levels in smokers.[10, 16, 17] Nonetheless, the benefit from decreased fibroids does not outweigh the substantial risks of smoking.

Diet also appears to influence fibroid risk. Women with diets rich in fruits and vegetables have a decreased risk of fibroids, and women with diets rich in red meats have an increased risk.[18] Consumption of alcohol, especially beer, also increases the risk of fibroids.[19] Caffeine has not been shown to affect risk.[19] No one has shown that changing our diet can change existing fibroids, however, or even prevent new ones. These studies show associations only.

Use of a *progestin-only contraceptive* such as Depo-Provera also appears to decrease the risk of having fibroids.[12] This has been best documented in African American women.

Body mass index (BMI; the relationship between weight and height) and weight appear to influence risk as well, with heavier women generally having greater risk.[20] However, no one has documented that losing weight helps with fibroids, although weight loss has many health benefits.

CHAPTER 2

What Are Uterine Fibroids?

Uterine fibroids are benign (meaning not cancerous or precancerous) growths in the uterine wall that often cause unpleasant and sometimes painful symptoms. To understand fibroids, you need to understand the structure of the normal uterus (fig. 2.1). The uterus is composed of two major layers. Most of the uterus is made of smooth muscle and is called the *myometrium*. The outermost portion of the myometrium is called the *serosa*. The lining of the uterus is a separate layer called the *endometrium*, which is not made of muscle. It is the innermost layer of the endometrium that is shed each month at the time of menstruation.

The terminology we use to describe the inside of the uterus can be confusing. The inside of the uterus is usually called the *endometrial* cavity or sometimes the *uterine cavity*. It is called the endometrial cavity because it is lined by the endometrium. Although drawings (including the ones in this book) typically show this as an open triangular space, in reality it is usually a potential space; most of the time the uterus is collapsed so that there is only a tiny amount of fluid separating the endometrium on the front side of the uterus from the endometrium on the back. This is why tests that place fluid inside the uterus are sometimes necessary to get a clear view of the endometrium.

The endometrium is also called the *mucosal surface* of the uterus. (The inside of other body organs, like the mouth, bowel or bladder, is also called the mucosal surface). We commonly use the term *submucosal* to refer to fibroids that are underneath ("sub-") the endometrium.

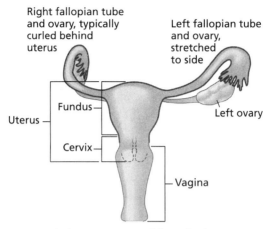

Whole organs, viewed from the front

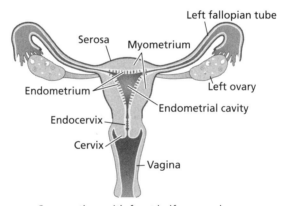

Cross section, with front half removed

Figure 2.1. The uterus is an organ that is composed predominantly of smooth muscle called myometrium. The thin layer of lining is called the endometrium. The outer layer of the muscle is called the serosa. The serosal layer is continuous with the lining of the pelvic and abdominal cavity (the *peritoneum*). Both fallopian tubes enter the endometrial cavity at the top. If you think of your body as the uterus with your arms out to the sides as fallopian tubes, the ovaries are tucked underneath your arms. The fallopian tubes can move like arms to pick up the egg and carry it into the uterus. They can be out to the side of the uterus, in front, but are most commonly behind the uterus. The cervix is the part of the uterus that goes into the vagina. It is the doughnut-shaped object at the top of the vagina that women can feel as they insert a tampon or diaphragm. There is no clear dividing line separating the cervix from the rest of the uterus; however, the cell types are very different when viewed under a microscope. The normal uterus is approximately the size of a fist.

The uterus is also thought of as consisting of the *fundus*, or top of the uterus, and the cervix. Most women are familiar with the cervix as the part of the uterus that protrudes into the vagina. The cervix is shaped like a doughnut and is located at the back of the vagina. The outer surface of the cervix contains types of cells that are very different from the cells making up the smooth muscle of the uterus. The inner lining of the cervix, called the *endocervix*, also differs from the lining of the uterus. It is important to know that there is no easily identified dividing line between the fundus and the cervix.

During pregnancy, the endometrium nourishes the pregnancy, and the muscle cells both divide (hyperplasia) and enlarge (hypertrophy) so that the pregnant uterus can grow. This process may have important implications for uterine fibroids. One theory of fibroid development suggests that fibroids are confused myometrial cells that act as if they are pregnant all the time.[1]

Each fibroid arises from a single smooth muscle cell in the uterus, and therefore fibroids are considered clonal tumors.[2,3] (A clone is a group of genetically identical cells; it does not have to be created by the cloning process we hear about in the news.) This process is unlike the formation of malignant tumors, in which one cell becomes abnormal and then spreads through the body. Many separate fibroids can form at the same time, each starting from a different cell.

This process of converting normal, smooth muscle cells into fibroid precursors (transformation) is probably very common. Studies have demonstrated that when you look carefully at the uteruses of women, more than 80 percent will have some evidence of fibroids.[4] When these microscopic single-cell fibroids begin to grow (forming a clone) and grow big enough to be felt and to cause symptoms (growth acceleration), the process of forming fibroids becomes medically significant.

There is a great variety of sizes and locations of fibroids (fig. 2.2). Fibroids that produce symptoms can be as small as a marble. The largest reported fibroid ever removed weighed more than 40 pounds.[5]

In most cases the metric system is used to measure fibroids. Therefore most reports talk about centimeters (cm) or millimeters (mm) instead of inches. There are 10 mm in each cm and 2.2 cm in each inch. So a 10-inch fibroid is exactly the same size as a 22-cm fibroid and a 220-mm one. It is critical to look at the units of measurement when discussing size! Most fibroids are not spherical, so most people report 3 measurements, the length, width, and depth—as in a

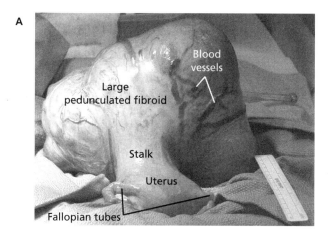

A

Blood vessels

Large pedunculated fibroid

Stalk

Uterus

Fallopian tubes

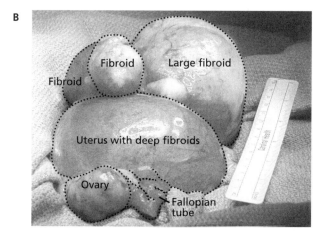

B

Fibroid

Large fibroid

Fibroid

Uterus with deep fibroids

Ovary

Fallopian tube

Figure 2.2. There is a huge range of sizes of fibroids. In fact, a fibroid the size of a dime on the inside of the uterus can cause substantial bleeding, and a large fibroid can reportedly have little symptoms. The fibroid may be much larger than the uterus, as seen in 2.2A. This is a pedunculated fibroid with the large stalk connecting the uterus (nearest to you) to the fibroid. Many women have multiple fibroids throughout the uterus, as seen in 2.2B. In this uterus it is difficult to distinguish the ovary (seen in the foreground with the fallopian tube) from multiple fibroids that fill the rest of the picture.

6.7 × 7.3 × 4.8 cm fibroid. If only one dimension is measured, it is usually the largest dimension.

Although size influences fibroid symptoms, location can be even more important. The relationship between the fibroid and the layers of the uterus is used to describe several different types of fibroids (fig. 2.3). For instance, fibroids that are distorting the endometrium or protruding into the endometrial cavity are called *submucosal* because they are below the mucosal surface. Fibroids protruding from the outer surface of the uterus, giving the uterus an irregular shape, are called *subserosal* fibroids. They distort the serosa, or outer layer of the uterus. *Intramural* fibroids are fibroids that are contained within the uterine wall. Generally, these fibroids enlarge the uterus but do not make it feel irregular.

Most fibroids are combinations of these various types. We are also not very precise in using these terms clinically. For example, many people will use the term *submucosal* to describe everything from a fibroid that is fully within the endometrial cavity to a fibroid that is mainly intramural but touching the endometrial surface. For these types of fibroids, the European Society of Hysteroscopy has provided a staging system that is quite useful.[6] The society has described three types of submucosal fibroids. A "Type 0" is contained entirely within the endometrial cavity. A "Type I" submucosal fibroid is one in which at least 50 percent of the fibroid is in the endometrial cavity. A "Type II" submucosal fibroid is a fibroid that intrudes into the endometrial cavity, but at least 50 percent of its bulk is within the uterine wall.

Other terms are sometimes used to describe the position of fibroids. *Pedunculated* means the fibroid has a stalk connecting it to the uterus. There are pedunculated submucosal fibroids (also known as Type 0) or pedunculated subserosal fibroids. Sometimes the term *exophytic* is used to describe subserosal fibroids significantly distorting the outer contour of the uterus.

Rather than using the European Society of Hysteroscopy classification for submucous fibroids, some reports attempt to describe the relationship between submucosal fibroids and the endometrium in words. However, because these descriptive terms have no clear definitions, they can cause significant confusion. They include "central fibroid," "fibroid abutting the endometrial cavity," and "fibroid distorting or bowing the endometrium."

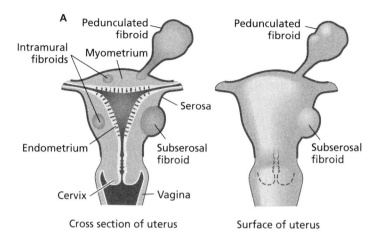

A

Pedunculated fibroid

Intramural fibroids

Myometrium

Endometrium

Cervix

Serosa

Subserosal fibroid

Vagina

Pedunculated fibroid

Subserosal fibroid

Cross section of uterus

Surface of uterus

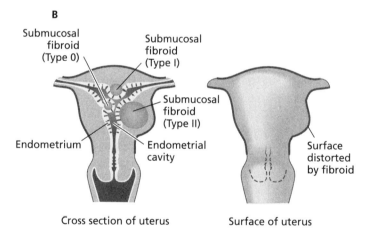

B

Submucosal fibroid (Type 0)

Submucosal fibroid (Type I)

Submucosal fibroid (Type II)

Endometrium

Endometrial cavity

Surface distorted by fibroid

Cross section of uterus

Surface of uterus

Figure 2.3. There are several important terms that describe the location of the fibroids. On the left side of each image you see the relationship of the fibroid to the endometrium, and on the right side a surface view is seen. As seen in 2.3A, subserosal fibroids are on the outer surface of the uterus and give the fibroid uterus its characteristic lumpy, bumpy feel. Pedunculated fibroids are on a stalk and are suspected clinically when the fibroid moves easily from place to place. Intramural fibroids are within the wall of the uterus. However, there are types of fibroids that can go from surface to surface; thus they can be intramural, submucosal, and subserosal all at the same time. In 2.3B the European Society of Hysteroscopy classification of submucosal fibroids is illustrated. Type 0 fibroids are contained entirely in the endometrium. With Type I fibroids, at least 50 percent of the fibroid's mass is in the endometrial cavity, and with Type II fibroids, at least 50 percent of the fibroid's mass is in the uterine wall.

Microscopic Facts about Fibroids

Fibroids are composed primarily of smooth muscle cells. The uterus, stomach, and bladder are all organs made of smooth muscle. Smooth muscle cells are arranged so that the organ can stretch, instead of being arranged in rigid units like the cells in skeletal muscle in arms and legs that are designed to "pull" in a particular direction.

Smooth muscle cells are long, stretched-out cells with a nucleus in the middle. They form interlacing bundles sort of like a woven basket. The thing that makes fibroids look different from normal uterine muscle is that they have an increased amount of extracellular matrix (ECM)—the collection of proteins and other substances found between cells that cause them to stick together, like the mortar or cement between bricks. This is also what makes the fibroids fibrous. ECM typically has an increased amount of collagen, the structural protein that is found in substances such as cartilage.[7] In addition, ECM serves as a storage site for a number of substances that appear to be important in terms of creating the symptoms of the fibroids. For many years ECM was thought only to provide support for cells, but research has shown that it is a very active, important part of any tissue or organ.

There is a significant amount of variability in the way fibroid tissue looks under the microscope. Some fibroids have many cells with small bands of ECM separating the bundles. In other fibroids there is a sea of ECM with a little island of fibroid cells (fig. 2.4). Nonetheless, it appears that ECM is an important part of fibroid biology.

Increased production of ECM causes problems in diseases other than fibroids. For example, scar tissue can form following surgery as the surgical site heals. It is likely an issue of balance; you want enough ECM to form after surgery to bring the tissue up to normal strength, but too much ECM can result in the formation of adhesions (abnormal tissue connecting two structures that are normally separated).

One such common problem is the formation of keloids, scars that are large, raised (hypertrophic), and darker in color (hyperpigmented) than regular scars. Because both fibroids and keloids are common in black women and both seem to be related to abnormal control of ECM formation, they may be related. In the future we may be able to approach fibrotic diseases (ones in which ECM production is increased or disordered) like keloids and fibroids with antifibrotic ther-

A

B

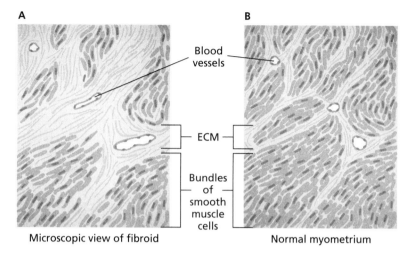

Blood vessels

ECM

Bundles of smooth muscle cells

Microscopic view of fibroid

Normal myometrium

Figure 2.4. Both fibroids (2.4A) and normal myometrium (2.4B) have nests of cells surrounded by extracellular matrix (ECM). However, as you can see in this example, this fibroid has a substantially increased amount of ECM separating bundles of muscle. The nucleus of each cell is seen as a black dash. You can see there is more room between these nuclei in the fibroid picture. The blood vessels travel through the tracts of ECM.

apies in the same way we are able to use similar hormonal therapies for different gynecologic diseases like fibroids and endometriosis.[7,8]

The endometrium (lining of the uterus) is also important in determining fibroid behavior (fig. 2.5). Because the endometrium is the layer that is shed during each menstrual cycle, there could not be any abnormal menstrual bleeding in women with fibroids without the endometrium. Specifically, it is the top two-thirds of the endometrium, called the *functional endometrium* (*endometrial functionalis*), that is shed each month. The bottommost third of the endometrium, the *base* (*basalis*), remains and directs the regeneration, or buildup, for the next cycle.

In women with fibroids, tissue from the endometrium typically looks normal under the microscope. Sometimes, however, over submucosal fibroids there is an unusual type of uterine lining that does not have the normal glandular structures. The presence of this abnormality, called *aglandular funtionalis* (functional endometrium with no glands), in women having bleeding difficulties is sometimes a clinical clue for their doctors to look more closely for a submucosal fibroid.[9] A second pattern of endometrium, termed *chronic endometritis*, can

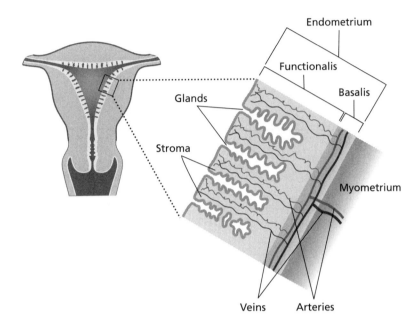

Figure 2.5. Although the endometrium as drawn in the book appears to be a simple layer, it is a very complicated structure. In fact, much more is known about the endometrium than about fibroids and myometrial smooth muscle. Two major types of structures make up the endometrium: the glands and the stroma. The glands are irregular pockets that project deep into the endometrium but completely line the inner surface of the uterus. The stroma is the denser supporting tissue where the blood vessels flow. At the end of each menstrual cycle the upper two-thirds of the endometrium, called the functionalis, or functioning part of the endometrium, falls off during menstruation. It is rebuilt from the basalis, or base.

also suggest that there may be a submucosal fibroid, although this pattern can also be associated with other problems such as pregnancy tissue not cleared from the uterus (retained products of conception) and various infections of the uterus. However, even when the lining looks normal under the microscope, examining the expression of particular molecules shows that the uterine lining in women with fibroids differs in important ways that make its function different from that of normal uterine lining.[10] These abnormalities may play a role in abnormal bleeding and pregnancy-related problems in women with fibroids.

Making Sense of Fibroid Variability

Clearly fibroids differ considerably in size, position, and appearance. Furthermore, under the microscope, there are even more differences. These differences in appearance probably lead to differences in the behavior of fibroids, but we do not understand the biology well enough to be able to categorize them. We are at the stage where all fibroids are fibroids, just like we used to refer to all cancers as cancer. When you treat cancers differently based on size, appearance, tissue of origin, cell type, and molecular expression, these differences are critical. Once we move beyond hysterectomy as a one-size-fits-all solution to fibroids, distinctions in size, position, and appearance will likely be important for treating fibroids. Once we understand these issues, we may be able to tell why some women have severe bleeding and other women with a similarly sized fibroid have no problem.

CHAPTER 3

Why We Are So Far Behind in Understanding and Treating Fibroids

It's a shame that there was never a Framingham Fibroid Project. For those of you who aren't familiar with the Framingham Heart Study, it was a landmark in our understanding of heart disease.[1] The founders of the study set out to follow a large group of men and women over time to see if they could understand why certain people developed heart disease.

All the information about heart disease that we take for granted today was not known when the study began. For instance, we didn't know that smoking and high blood pressure increase the risk of heart disease and that exercise decreases the risk.

Medical research works this way: The first step is to understand that high blood pressure (for example) and heart disease are related. High blood pressure may or may not cause heart disease, but they are associated. Once you have identified the association, you can find out whether changing the factor helps to prevent disease. If high blood pressure is related to heart disease, can you prevent heart attacks by better controlling blood pressure?

It seems so clear now, but it was not clear in the 1960s, when my grandfather was in his early fifties and had already had a heart attack. He changed to a less "stressful" job, but there were no medications to offer him to control his blood pressure and no reason to advise him to stop smoking. He died in his early fifties after several heart attacks and strokes. Today his doctors would have aggressively controlled his blood pressure and encouraged weight loss, smoking cessation, and exercise.

Thus, once you understand association, you can start to design potential interventions and test them to find out whether they reduce disease. We are not even at this step with fibroids. Women often ask:

> "What can I do to prevent having the same problems with fibroids that my mother had?"

> "What can I do to prevent my small fibroids from growing and causing me problems?"

> "Now that I have undergone surgery (or another therapy), what can I do to prevent having further problems?"

Currently the only answer we have to these questions is "We don't know." From our understanding of epidemiology (epidemiology is the study of why some people in a particular population get a disease and ways to prevent disease) and from clinical studies (which involve patients), we have some promising clues regarding what factors influence the need for additional surgeries following an initial surgery or procedure. However, we need more studies to find out whether lifestyle interventions or dietary changes can lead to prevention strategies for fibroid tumors.

The process of discovering associations comes not only from epidemiologic and clinical work but also from basic or laboratory science. We call this, in medicine, the study of pathophysiology of the disease: a combination of physiology (how the body systems work normally) and pathology (the process by which disease occurs). As I mentioned in the Introduction, much more is known about the smooth muscle cells that line the arteries or veins in our bodies than about the smooth muscle cells of the uterus. Thus, we understand the biology of atherosclerosis ("hardening of the arteries") better than the reasons for fibroid formation. We know that an atherosclerotic plaque has something to do with diet (intake of cholesterol-rich foods), genetics (differences in individuals' ability to clear cholesterol from the bloodstream), and exercise (changing the nervous system's input into the constriction of blood vessels).

In my grandfather's case, a better understanding of biology would have led to testing his cholesterol and potentially prescribing a drug to bring his cholesterol levels down. If the levels were very high, the doctors may have advised him to get genetic testing to see whether he had a rare type of lipid disorder, and, if so, they may have recommended genetic testing for my mother (his daughter) and perhaps for me, as well. They might have recommended taking a baby aspirin daily to change the interaction of blood platelets with the wall of the arteries and decrease the risk of clotting, which can lead to a heart attack. We don't have any of these kinds of interventions for fibroids.

The final way in which research is useful is that it can lead to revolutionary treatments because of new understanding of disease. We are currently seeing this change in cancer treatment. The earliest cancer treatments focused on killing all rapidly dividing cells. This approach can be very effective for many cancers but is limited by side effects: nausea, vomiting, and diarrhea (due to killing the rapidly dividing cells lining the gut) and hair loss (because hair follicles are rapidly dividing cells). By understanding why different cancers develop, doctors were first able to develop specific chemotherapy regimens that dealt with specific kinds of cancers: cancer of the ovary is treated differently than lung cancer.

Now we are at the point where biology has revolutionized cancer treatment. First, there is a specific treatment, Gleevec (imatinib mesylate), that was developed by understanding basic biology.[2] Researchers in Philadelphia first noted that chronic myelogenous leukemia (CML, a blood cell cancer) is associated with a specific pattern of broken chromosomes in which part of chromosome 9 becomes attached to chromosome 22. This became known as the Philadelphia chromosome and was found in most people with CML. Further research discovered that a new protein was produced when this chromosome break took place. This new protein is called a fusion protein, since part of the BCR protein on chromosome 22 is fused with the ABL protein from chromosome 9. The BCR-ABL protein made a superactive enzyme that was working all the time and led to the cancerous change of these white blood cells.

For many years, CML was treated by conventional chemotherapy. But then researchers studied the BCR-ABL enzyme and designed a specific inhibitor for it: a protein that binds to the working site of the enzyme and blocks it. The inhibitor is imatinib mesylate and is a major advance over previous therapies because it works specifically in the cancer cells, since they are the only ones that have the chromosome breaks to create this abnormal enzyme. Normal cells are not affected by imatinib mesylate, so the side effects are minimized.

Advanced scientific techniques may also help us pick the most effective treatments for each individual. Traditionally, to pick a treatment for cancer we relied on clinical predictors (such as a woman's age, race, and menopausal status), histological predictors (the type and appearance of the tumor's cells), and staging (how far the tumor has spread throughout the body) to help determine how aggressive the tumor was and estimate the odds of when, or if, the tumors would recur. With this approach, some women got more aggressive treatment than they needed (experiencing the side effects with no benefit), and other women did not receive additional therapy that would have benefited them.

With a new genetic technique called a gene chip (technically a DNA microarray), hundreds of genes can be examined at once by finding the pieces of DNA on a glass slide that match the DNA of the tumor. This technique is much more powerful than testing approximately a dozen histological or clinical factors. Studies are now able to identify particular genes that lead to bad outcomes and thus identify women who need specific treatment or more aggressive treatment.[3]

We need tools like gene chips to better manage diseases like fibroids. Tools such as this might allow us to predict which women will have pregnancy problems related to their fibroids and which women will need a repeat surgery soon after undergoing a myomectomy.

Because we concentrated on surgically taking fibroids out for so many years rather than discovering the underlying biology, we also lack some conventional tools for studying fibroids. Having animal models of disease is useful in understanding the role of specific hormones or environmental factors or even in testing new therapies. It is easier to see whether cigarette smoke causes lung cancer by exposing rats or mice to tar and nicotine than to separate out all of the personal influences of people who have lung cancer and smoke. Similarly, animals with diabetes can be treated with investigational drugs to see whether their blood sugar becomes normal or whether they develop diabetic problems with their eyes at the same rate as animals not receiving the drugs.

Mice that develop specific diseases are especially helpful to researchers these days. Mice are small and thus more easily housed and inexpensive to feed and maintain than rats, guinea pigs, or monkeys. Also, we know more about the genetics of mice than that of any other species and have discovered that many genes are similar from one species to another and perform similar tasks. This can help us assess the role that specific genes play in the process of fibroid formation. If we had a mouse model for fibroids, we could "knock out" (inactivate or delete) a gene thought to play an important role to see whether the fibroids disappeared.

The two major animal models we have are a rat model, which develops fibroid lesions spontaneously as a result of a gene mutation (the Eker rat model), and a guinea pig model, which develops fibroids after long-term exposure to high levels of estrogen and progesterone. Both of these models are more costly than mice and are less useful for studying the genetics of disease.

Fibroid treatment is stuck in the 1960s era of treatment. Why? Cynics would suggest that because fibroids are a disease that specifically affects women and particularly black women, it has not been viewed as important. Although there may be issues of sexism and racism in the scientific study of fibroids, social and cultural trends have changed our attitudes toward this disease.

Changes in women's lifestyles have had a major impact on the disease. First, our feeling about hysterectomy has markedly changed over the years. Before minimally invasive options were available, hysterectomy provided a complete solution. In the 1950s and 1960s the treatment of fibroids by hysterectomy put fibroids ahead of heart attacks in terms of available treatment options. The fact that good contraception was not widely available to women also led some women to seek hysterectomy, whereas today they would elect to use birth control pills or an IUD or undergo a tubal ligation.

The pattern of having children later in life has also had a dramatic impact on the choice of therapies. When women had their children in their twenties and early thirties and then developed fibroids in their forties, moving on to hysterectomy was a more acceptable solution. Now many more women develop fibroids before their childbearing is completed or, in many cases, even started. Although minimally invasive therapies were originally developed to allow continued childbearing, the advantage of the quick recovery has led to a more widespread use of them.

The changing importance of women economically has also aided the search for better interventions for uterine fibroids. Although a mother missing two days a month caring for her children because of heavy menses is no less important than an executive missing two days a month at the office, our society has an easier time estimating the costs to society in the latter situation. Likewise, being away from work for 6 to 8 weeks following a hysterectomy is more of an economic issue in an era in which many women are the primary or sole wage earners for the family.

In fact, accurately capturing all the costs attributable to uterine fibroids will help us move toward more, and more effective, innovative therapies. When deciding whether or not to launch a new product, companies typically look at the amount currently spent for other treatments. The economics of fibroids has chiefly been discussed in terms of the health care costs of hysterectomy. This in itself is a huge amount of money. According to a recent estimate, in the United States, more than $2 billion every year is spent on hospitalization costs due to uterine fibroids alone.[4] Additionally, one study estimates that the health care costs due to uterine fibroids are more than $4,600 per woman per year.[5]

When you incorporate all the costs of fibroids, however, the total is even more significant:

- The costs of myomectomy, uterine artery embolization (UAE), and other minimally invasive therapies
- The costs of birth control pills and other hormonal treatments to control bleeding
- The costs of tampons, pads, and the adult diapers many women require to contain the bleeding
- The costs of alternative and complementary therapies
- The cost of doing nothing (for many women this means missing work or working less productively during their period)

Many women are so used to adjusting their lives around their periods that they don't even see this accommodation as a problem. One woman said she worked from home for the first three days of her period, but she said this routine was fine, since her job was flexible. However, when I asked her whether she would see it as a problem if she had such bad diarrhea she had to stay home regularly, the importance was clear.

CHAPTER 4

The Endocrinology
of the Uterus

The endocrine system is the system of hormones that affect many body functions. Hormones are produced in many different organs (termed *endocrine organs*) and circulate throughout the body in the bloodstream to cause many different body changes. The entire reproductive system starts in the brain in both men and women. In the part of the brain called the hypothalamus, a small protein hormone called gonadotropin-releasing hormone (GnRH) is produced by specialized nerve cells. These nerve cells release a burst of GnRH approximately once an hour. This intermittent or pulsatile (pulse-like) release of GnRH is critical to reproductive function. Having either too little or too much GnRH shuts down the entire system.

The Role of the Hypothalamus and Pituitary in Reproduction

Most of the GnRH never gets out into the body circulation. Instead, it travels just a short distance to another part of the brain called the pituitary. A large net of blood vessels arises in the hypothalamus and leads to the pituitary. The pituitary gland hangs down slightly from the brain and is located in the region right behind the bridge of the nose. The pituitary gland has been called the master gland because it controls so many important bodily functions. The GnRH that is released in a pulse is directed through this net of blood vessels to the pituitary. Together, the pituitary and the hypothalamus control reproduction.

The anterior, or frontal, part of the pituitary has specialized cells that release several specific body-control hormones. The cells we are most interested in are the gonadotropes. They produce the hormones that control the gonads (in women, the ovaries; in men, the testes). The two hormones that the gonadotropes release are gonadotrophins, or growth hormones for the gonads: follicle-stimulating hormone (FSH) and luteinizing hormone (LH). FSH and LH are secreted in increased quantities at the time of puberty, which leads to the development of the sexually mature ovaries and testes. The names of these hormones come from their function in women, but they carry out similar functions in both men and women.

In the ovary, FSH and LH play different roles (fig. 4.1). FSH dominates during the first half of the menstrual cycle, as the ovarian follicle forms. The follicle is the clear fluid-filled space where the egg grows and matures. Therefore, FSH is in many ways the egg-stimulating hormone. FSH also controls the production of the major female hormone estrogen, which is made as the egg develops. Estrogen goes back to the brain to suppress FSH production as the egg matures. From the point of view of the uterus, however, estrogen's most important task is to cause the uterine lining (and potentially the fibroids) to grow and thicken in preparation for the implantation of the egg.

The name luteinizing hormone comes from the fact that after ovulation LH stimulates the production of the corpus luteum. *Corpus luteum* means "yellow body" in Latin; it is a yellowish part of the ovary where cholesterol (typically yellow in color) is converted to progesterone following ovulation.

An initial surge of LH first triggers release of the egg. The corpus luteum is then formed after the egg follicle has ruptured and released the egg. Blood vessels grow into this space delivering cholesterol from the bloodstream, and the enzymes stimulated there convert cholesterol in the blood to the steroid hormone progesterone. Thus, LH plays the dominant role in the second half of the menstrual cycle, after the egg is released, stimulating and maintaining the production of the hormone progesterone.

When progesterone is released after ovulation, it functions to organize the uterine lining and stabilize it so that it can fall off in an orderly fashion if pregnancy does not occur that cycle. Progesterone

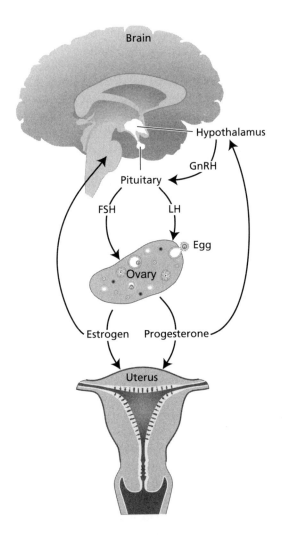

Figure 4.1. The reproductive system is controlled by the hypothalamus and pituitary. In women the ovary and the uterus also play important roles. GnRH is the hormone that is released from the hypothalamus in a pulse approximately once an hour. This hormone flows directly to the pituitary, which hangs down from the brain and secretes important hormones, including FSH and LH. FSH and LH work on the ovary to cause production both of mature eggs and of the hormones estrogen and progesterone. These hormones, in turn, go to the uterus to prepare it for pregnancy or to set up the cyclic changes of menstruation if pregnancy doesn't occur. The ovarian hormones provide feedback to the brain to regulate the system. This is called "negative" feedback because the ovarian hormones lead to a decrease in the brain hormones.

is also the major influence on preparing the uterus for a pregnancy (thus its name, from "pro-gestation"). These hormones play analogous roles in men: FSH is the major control for sperm production, and LH is the major control for testosterone production.

This system is very finely tuned. Both the amount of GnRH released and the frequency with which it is released send a signal to the pituitary to influence the proportion of FSH to be made relative to the amount of LH. Therefore, the system is easily shut down if the precise sequence of signaling is not maintained. If the pulse system of GnRH is disrupted so that GnRH is continually present, the system will shut down. This mechanism can be exploited by drugs, as we will see in a later chapter.

There are several other hypothalamic and pituitary hormones that we will discuss later which do not act to stimulate the ovary. These hormones include prolactin and vasopressin.

Steroid Hormones

The gonadal steroid hormones (estrogen, progesterone, and testosterone) also act on the brain, letting it know that the stimulation has been successful. This is called negative feedback because the hormones lead to the repression of the stimulating hormones. These steroid hormones also affect many body tissues, including breasts, bone, hair follicles, and muscle.

Typically when people hear the term *steroid hormones*, they think about the anabolic steroids athletes use to bulk up. These "steroids" are only a small part of this important class of hormones. The category is based on their molecular structure, which helps them pass easily into cells.

In women, the uterus is quiescent or quiet (as it is before puberty) until stimulated by estrogen and progesterone. Most of the study of uterine function has concentrated on the endometrium, the thin layer of uterine lining that is shed during menstruation and is transformed into the bed for the placenta during pregnancy. In the endometrium, as mentioned earlier, estrogen tends to build up the lining, and progesterone organizes it in preparation for menstruation or pregnancy. Estrogen and progesterone also affect the muscle layer where fibroids arise. It is less clear how this part of the system works.

It is not clear that the uterus sends hormonal signals back to the rest of the reproductive system, but there is evidence of at least some communication from the uterus to the ovary. Several studies have shown that having a tubal ligation or a hysterectomy while leaving the ovaries in place decreases the risk of ovarian cancer.[1,2]

There are also fine points to the action of these steroid hormones in target tissues like fibroids but also in the brain, bone, and breast. Steroid hormones can easily pass through the cell membrane and carry out their action in the nucleus of the cell, the control center where the DNA directs the action (fig. 4.2). The key to understanding the action of these hormones is that they bind with proteins called receptors; it is the hormone-receptor complex that brings about the changes by binding to DNA. Hormones and receptors fit together like locks and keys. The analogy is apt. You can have an office-specific key as well as a pass key that fits all the locks in the office; similarly, different hormone-receptor combinations can give different results. You can also have a key that fits into the keyhole but does not open the door; in the language of hormones this "key" is called a hormone blocker or antagonist.

The first level of control for steroid hormone action is the exact hormone present—in other words, which key is used. For estrogen, there are several different natural estrogens, with estradiol being the most common estrogen in women with fibroids. There are also many different formulations of estrogen supplements—both natural estrogens from plants or animals and synthetic estrogens—all of which need to interact with receptors to carry out their action. The exact estrogen used can be important in determining the result.

A special class of drug compounds commonly called "designer estrogens," but more correctly termed *selective estrogen receptor modulators* (SERMs), have been designed to perform special jobs. One ideal role for a SERM is to act like an estrogen at the sites in the body where estrogen is beneficial (like the brain and bone) but to act like an estrogen blocker at the breast to decrease the risk of breast cancer. All hormones have some mixture in their action, which is why women may respond differently to different compounds. Progesterone-like substances are termed *progestins*. Progesterone is far and away the most important natural compound, but there are a number of synthetic progestins like medroxyprogesterone acetate (used in hormone replacement) and norethindrone and levonorgestrel (used

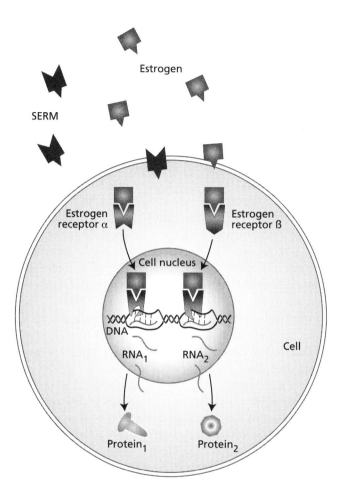

Figure 4.2. Steroid hormones such as estrogen, progesterone, and testosterone work in the nucleus of the cell. They easily pass through cell membranes and bind to receptors in the cells. Different hormones and different types of receptors can bind to DNA in slightly different ways to turn on specific proteins. In this illustration both estrogen and a selective estrogen receptor modulator (SERM, such as tamoxifen) go easily from the bloodstream (in the upper left) into the cell and on into the nucleus. Although in this diagram it is estrogen that is interacting with both the alpha and beta estrogen receptors to produce two different RNAs and thus two different proteins, the SERM could also interact with each and have a different effect on the cell.

for contraceptives). The hormone can be changed to make it easier to use—for example, so that it can be taken as a pill instead of as a shot or so that doses don't need to be given so frequently—but altering the hormone may also change its action.

There are compounds analogous to SERMs for progesterone, termed *selective progesterone receptor modulators* (PRMs or SPRMs), but these are further behind in commercial development.[3,4] Two PRMs that are undergoing clinical trials for the treatment of uterine fibroids are Asoprisnil (previously called J867) and Proellix (previously called Progenta).

Androgens are thought of as male hormones, but they are present in women, too. Both the ovaries and the adrenal gland (another endocrine gland, located next to the kidney) make androgens that are present in the circulation. Women have low levels of testosterone and other natural androgens, including androstenedione and dehydroepiandrosterone (DHEA), compared with men, but these hormones play important roles.

Androgens act on hair follicles and likely have a role in sex drive and mood. Importantly, androgens are used to make estrogens. In fact, the ovarian follicle makes androgens and converts them to estrogens using an enzyme called aromatase. This is why women who don't ovulate can have androgenic side effects like acne and increased body and facial hair. Body fat also "aromatizes" androgens to estrogens, which is why heavier women have higher levels of estrogen.

There are also synthetic androgens we use for treatment of gynecologic disease. The most common one used in women is danazol, which is primarily used for the treatment of endometriosis.

Although we divide steroid hormones into the categories of estrogen, progestin, and androgen, some molecules will fit into more than one category. Different parts of the steroid molecules are like different notches on the key. Many synthetic progestins have androgen-like effects and thus cause androgenic side effects like acne and increased hair growth. Also, there are molecules like tibolone that work like an estrogen and a progestin (two keys in one!).

The dose or amount of the steroid hormone is also important in determining its action. Just as with any medication, a high dose will likely cause different effects and side effects than a low dose of the same compound.

Duration of exposure to steroid hormones is also important. When you take an antibiotic to treat a urinary tract infection and the directions are to take a tablet twice a day for 10 days, you won't have the same chance of curing the infection if you take all 20 at one time. This is a special issue for the endometrium and its exposure to progestins: you often need a lower dose longer to get the desired effect.

Finally, the route of delivery makes a difference in hormonal action. Pills or other kinds of oral medications enter the body through the digestive tract and reach the liver in very high concentrations compared with medication delivered by a patch, which is absorbed by the skin (the blood vessels from the gut are routed through the liver). Because the liver makes factors that affect blood clotting, oral preparations are more likely to cause blood clots as a side effect.

There is also a difference between systemic delivery (the medication is delivered through the whole body to reach the place where it is really needed) and local or targeted delivery (the highest concentration is where you want it to be). Using a medicated intrauterine device (IUD) or vaginal delivery of medication provides targeted delivery for the uterus.

The kind of receptor (the lock) in a tissue also contributes to the way steroid hormones act. There are two different kinds of receptors for estrogen (ER-α and ERβ) and progesterone (PR A and PR B). Fibroids have both different amounts and different ratios of these receptors than normal myometrium.[5–7] Moreover, many steroid hormone receptors work in pairs. So, for example, with the progesterone receptor, 3 combinations are possible: PR A–PR A, PR A–PR B, and PR B–PR B.

Finally, each tissue in the body has specific factors that regulate steroid hormone action. Not only does the breast potentially have a different mix of estrogen and progesterone receptors than does bone, but all kinds of other tissue-specific factors also come into play. The DNA folding may make it easy for hormones to stimulate RNA production, or it may have other molecules that block these binding sites. There are a number of other terms like *promoters*, *repressors*, and *coactivators* that describe molecules that specific cells may have that make hormone-stimulated RNA synthesis (production) easier or harder.

The complexity of the hormone system thus makes it impossible to say, for example, that progestins cause fibroids to shrink. To adequately determine whether this is the case, many questions need to be asked: what specific progestin, what dose, for how long, in a pill or in an IUD, and so on. Understanding the biology does not always lead to simple answers.

Protein Hormones

In addition to steroid hormones like estrogen and progesterone, the endocrine system produces a number of protein hormones such as insulin, the hormone that is lacking in Type I diabetes, and growth hormone, too little of which results in dwarfism and too much causes a disease called acromegaly. FSH and LH belong to this class of hormones.

We don't know a lot about how protein hormones influence uterine fibroids, but proteins do appear to influence fibroid biology in a few areas. Protein hormones may provide new targets for innovative therapies in the future.

Proteins are large, bulky molecules that do not easily pass into the cell. They exert their influence on the cell by binding to receptors (other proteins that are the lock to the hormone's key) on the outside of the cell (fig. 4.3). The binding of the hormone to the receptor causes new small molecules to be formed inside the cell that carry out its action. These intracellular molecules are called second messengers and start a cascade of events that lead to specific genes being turned on in the nucleus.

Growth Factors

Growth factors are smaller proteins (also called peptides) that can carry out actions inside and between the cells. In fibroid research several different families of growth factors have been identified as important: angiogenic growth factors, fibrotic growth factors, and insulin-like growth factors.

Angiogenic growth factors influence the formation or function of blood vessels. The best-described angiogenic growth factor in fibroid biology is basic fibroblast growth factor (bFGF). This growth factor is overproduced in fibroids, and the protein is stored in the extracellular matrix (ECM).[8] It also appears that the receptor for bFGF in the endometrium is not regulated correctly.[9] Thus, abnormalities of the

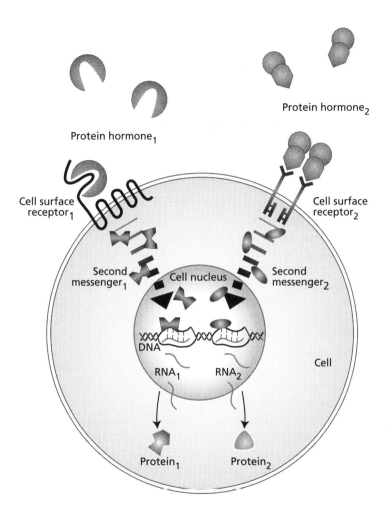

Figure 4.3. Protein hormones work differently than steroid hormones. Proteins are large bulky molecules and therefore cannot easily get inside cells. Therefore, they bind to their receptors on the cell surface. This leads to activation and production of new factors inside the cell that are classically termed "second messenger" molecules. Different molecules bind to different receptor types and can stimulate different signaling pathways. There are several different types of cell surface receptors. The receptor illustrated on the left is similar to the receptor for hormones such as LH and FSH, and the receptor on the right is similar to the type of receptor insulin uses. Protein hormones also lead to the production of new RNAs and proteins through the actions of the second messengers.

bFGF system may be responsible for abnormal menstrual bleeding with fibroids.

Fibrotic growth factors influence the formation of the ECM and are another major growth factor family. These hormones are important in normal wound healing, but when they lead to the production of too much ECM, scar tissue and conditions such as fibroids can form. Transforming growth factor beta (TGF-ß) is the best studied of the fibrotic factors.[10–12] There are several subtypes of TGF-ßs and several different receptors. Some are distinctly abnormal in the majority of women with fibroids.

Additional components of the fibrotic factor pathway appear to be abnormally regulated in leiomyomas. Related molecules like Smads (molecules that transmit the signals generated by TGF-ßs), matrix metaloproteinases (MMPs, which are enzymes that break down ECM), and tissue inhibitors of metaloproteinases (TIMPs, which are substances that keep MMPs inactive) all are involved in the fibrotic biology of fibroids.[13–15] Particular ECM proteins, including collagens type 1 and III and dermatopontin, are also important.[16,17]

Finally, the insulin-like growth factor (IGF) system likely is also important in fibroid biology.[18–20] Again, as with the TGF-ß family, there are several IGFs and several IGF binding proteins (IGFBPs) that keep the factors inactive, as well as multiple receptors. These small molecules have some insulin-like action.

Most of the currently available medical therapies come from the knowledge (gained through basic science experiments) that fibroids and normal myometrium respond differently to estrogen and progesterone or have different susceptibility to these hormones. Understanding other biological differences between myometrium and fibroids gives us prospects for new treatments that exploit these differences. Thus, understanding growth factors may lead to new treatments with fewer side effects in the future.

CHAPTER 5

Why Do Fibroids Form?

We do not know why fibroids form. Furthermore, although we know some of the hormones important for fibroids, we don't understand how these hormonal influences lead to the abnormal bleeding that characterizes this disease. Originally, we simplistically assumed that women with uterine fibroids had an enlarged endometrial cavity and therefore this larger surface caused increased bleeding at the time of menstruation. While increased surface area may play a role, we want to explore all the possible causes. In this chapter we will examine a number of theories that may influence fibroid formation, growth, and symptoms.

Genetic Causes of Fibroids

One major theory is that some women are genetically predisposed to form fibroids. We see many families in which women in every generation are affected by fibroids. In some families, however, a woman's maternal relatives do not have fibroids, but the aunts and cousins on her father's side of the family have significant problems with fibroids. Thus, it appears you may inherit an increased risk of fibroids from either your mother or your father. (This situation raises the intriguing and unanswered question of what these genes do in the men who inherit the gene.)

Why would a gene that produces something bad like fibroids be passed on? It turns out that many genes that today produce something bad may, in the past, have given our ancestors a benefit and thus a survival advantage. The factors that lead to fibroid formation may be adaptive just like the mutation in the hemoglobin gene that causes sickle cell disease also protects against malaria.

In the era when many women died in childbirth and women rarely lived to their forties, even if women had a genetic predisposition to form fibroids, few women did. Furthermore, the few women who did develop fibroids had fewer symptoms if they were frequently pregnant or breast-feeding. If the same gene that causes fibroids also did something good such as defending against infectious disease or leading to stronger, healthier babies or more milk production following pregnancy, it passed on a selective advantage to women and their babies for many generations. Only in the modern era did the gene provide a disadvantage in women who develop fibroids.

It is likely that there are, indeed, many different kinds of fibroids resulting from many different genes. For this reason we say fibroids are a phenotype or expression of disease that results from many different genotypes or different root causes. (This topic is discussed in detail in Chapter 17, on genetics.)

Environmental Causes of Fibroids

Environmental factors either by themselves or by interacting with genes may influence fibroid formation or growth. Studies suggest that diet, smoking, and various forms of contraception influence the risk of fibroids. Scientists have also been actively searching to see whether various chemicals in the environment influence fibroid risk. These factors may cause fibroids to form or cause preexisting fibroids to grow.

Alternatively, new environmental factors may cause expression of genes present for many generations that previously had been silent. Of particular concern are pesticides or agents in the environment that have estrogen-like action, termed *xenoestrogens.*

Steroid Hormones

What is clear is that fibroids respond to the ovarian steroid hormones estrogen and progesterone. Most of the literature written about fibroids cites only estrogen as an important influence, but there is evidence that progesterone may be equally or perhaps even more important.

The fact that women do not develop fibroids until they have completed puberty and that fibroids typically shrink at the time of menopause supports this dependence on steroid hormones. Another line of reasoning to support this theory is that most effective medical treatments for fibroids, such as gonadotropin-releasing hormone (GnRH) agonists, decrease the levels of both estrogen and progesterone. As we will see in later chapters, there are times when progesterone seems to be the important hormone. However, all women have significant exposure to estrogen and progesterone, but not all women develop fibroids. Thus, there are other critical influences.

Fibroids as a Disease of Fibrosis

There is also evidence that fibroids may be characterized as a disease of abnormal fibrosis.[1,2] Other disease processes, such as the formation of keloids, result when the body produces too much extracellular matrix (ECM) in a disordered fashion. There are some parallels in the biology of uterine fibroids and that of keloids, which may explain why black women (who are particularly affected by fibroids) are at increased risk for keloids, also.

Fibroids as a Disease of Abnormal Blood Vessels

There is evidence that goes back almost a hundred years that the blood vessels in the fibroid uterus are abnormal.[3,4] The original studies were done by injecting the uterine blood vessels with a latexlike substance after hysterectomy. These studies determined that there was an increased number of arteries and veins in the uterus. The process of forming new blood vessels is termed *angiogenesis*. Angiogenesis is an abnormal occurrence in most organs, such as in the eye when, under the influence of diabetes, new blood vessels are formed and interfere with vision. It is also an important factor in most cancers. However, the uterus and the ovaries are different from most other organs, as new blood vessel formation occurs every month in the uterus and ovaries with the start of a new menstrual cycle. A number of angiogenic growth factors (factors that stimulate new blood vessel formation) are found in increased amounts in fibroids. The most commonly reported angiogenic growth factor is basic fibroblast growth factor (bFGF), as we discussed in Chapter 4. It is likely that many other angiogenic factors are important in the fibroid uterus.[5]

The latex injection studies also showed what was termed *venule ectasia*. This means that the veins were more floppy and had an increased capacity.

Why does venule ectasia occur? The original theory was that the physical compression of the fibroids blocked the return of blood through the veins, just as during pregnancy the pregnant uterus presses on the blood vessels so that there is swelling of the legs and formation of varicose veins.[6] However, given that women move freely and the uterus moves with a woman's movement, this is unlikely to be the full explanation.

It is likely that venule ectasia too has a molecular explanation.[7] Perhaps the veins in the fibroid uterus have an abnormal structure. Alternatively, the vessels could be structurally normal yet the surrounding abnormal ECM causes ectasia by allowing the blood vessels to stretch abnormally or by preventing the blood vessels from contracting and clotting off following menstruation.

Fibroids as a Disease of Altered Menstruation Patterns

For most of history, women spent most of their short lives pregnant or breast-feeding, and thus the pattern of monthly menstruation is relatively new.[8] The role of constant menstrual cyclicity brought about by effective birth control may play a role in the formation of uterine fibroids as well as other gynecologic diseases. We think of fibroids as static lumps of tissue, but they are constantly being remodeled when certain genes are turned on (and others turned off) every month based on the hormonal fluxes of the normal menstrual cycle.[7]

A theory that I call my "broken light bulb" hypothesis is that this constant flux may be responsible for inducing mistakes that result in fibroid formation or growth. Just as you are more likely to get a light bulb filament to burst by rapidly and repeatedly turning the switch off and on and making the filament heat and cool down, the system may be stressed by the rapid, repetitive change of gene transcription. Having 13 periods a year for up to 40 years provides many opportunities for mistakes.

Alternatively, since women with fibroids often report having periods that are painful or heavy (or both) from a young age, there has been some speculation that ischemia, or loss of blood supply during menstruation, may cause an injury that leads to fibroid formation.[1] Thus, menstrual cyclicity and genetic or environmental factors causing injury may be the initial problem, and fibroids are the end result of damage. If this is indeed the case, preventing the cause of painful periods in adolescence may decrease fibroid formation in mature women, a true win-win situation.

Previously I mentioned the theory that fibroids are myometrium that "thinks" it is pregnant all the time.[9] One reason for this theory is that the genes expressed in the myometrium of pregnancy are similar to the genes turned on in fibroids compared with the normal myometrium.[9,10] There is also some evidence that the process of involution (going back to normal size) following pregnancy gets rid of small fibroids, and this may be why having pregnancies protects against the development of fibroids.[11] Thus the fact that modern women have fewer pregnancies may cause an increase in fibroids that are clinically detected.

These theories are not necessarily mutually exclusive. Since fibroids may arise from different causes, some of these theories may apply only to certain individuals. Alternatively, many may apply in other instances. For example, a genetic reason for sensitivity to steroid hormones may interact with an environmental trigger. It is important to keep our mind open to new explanations for fibroid formation, since this may lead to new pathways to treatment.

CHAPTER 6

Diagnosis: How Do I Know That I Have Fibroids?

Question 1. How do I know that I have fibroids?

A diagnosis of fibroids is typically suspected based on symptoms the woman describes or when a doctor finds an enlarged, irregular uterus during a pelvic examination. A pelvic ultrasound is usually done to confirm the diagnosis of fibroids and to exclude other, more worrisome problems, such as ovarian cancer. If there is an enlarged but smooth uterus, excluding the possibility that the woman might be pregnant is important. Most, but not all, fibroids are seen during an ultrasound exam, and ultrasound is an excellent tool for seeing the ovaries.

Ultrasound is relatively inexpensive, comfortable for patients, and widely available and involves no exposure to X-rays. Generally a transvaginal ultrasound (in which the ultrasound transducer is placed in the vagina) gives the best view of the fibroids because the fibroids are in the middle of the pelvis and right next to the vagina. However, some fibroids are so large they reach up outside the pelvis, and in this case transabdominal ultrasound is used (the transducer is placed against the stomach). This approach usually requires the woman to have a full bladder (which acts as a window to see through) and thus can take more time to prepare for and can be slightly uncomfortable.

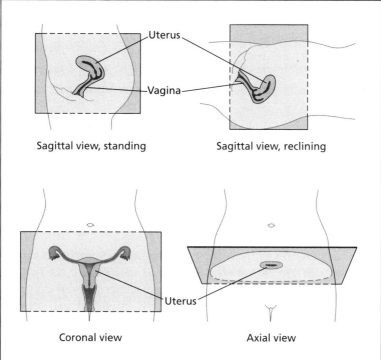

Sagittal view, standing   Sagittal view, reclining

Coronal view   Axial view

Understanding the Terminology of Diagnostic Imaging
Understanding the terms *sagittal, axial,* and *coronal* is vital when you are viewing anatomic images. A sagittal scan employs a "sideways view." Thus the position of the uterus may be different depending on whether the woman is standing or reclining. Most of the images in this book have the woman in the standing orientation for images. Typically the belly is on the left side of the image, and the back is on the right. An axial scan shows a horizontal section of the same standing woman when viewed from the top. The belly is at the top of the picture, and the spine and buttocks are at the bottom. A coronal scan looks at a standing person who is facing you, and images go from the anterior abdomen through the back. Because it is like looking in a mirror, the right side is depicted on the left side of the image.

Ultrasounds are not as good for seeing the inside of the uterus and finding small submucosal fibroids or endometrial polyps, the other structural lesions often found inside the uterus. Although diagrams of the uterus in this book show the endometrial cavity open, in reality it is usually collapsed so that the endometrium in the front of the uterus is touching the endometrium in the back. By ultrasound, however, we can determine the "thickness" of the endometrium, referred to as the endometrial stripe, by measuring from the base of one side of the endometrial stripe to the base of the other; however, submucosal fibroids can hide in this space (fig. 6.1). You can visualize how this happens by taking a small piece of tissue, crumpling it up, and putting it between your hands as you touch your palms together. When your hands are touching, you cannot see anything inside; only when you separate your hands at the wrists so that just your fingertips touch do you see the mass hiding inside.

Measuring the endometrial stripe has been very useful in screening postmenopausal women for endometrial cancer because the normal lining in postmenopausal women is thin. It is less useful in premenopausal women, since the normal lining is thicker and varies throughout the menstrual cycle.

A technique that opens up the endometrial cavity, so that the endometrium can be differentiated from structural lesions of the uterus, is often required to find these small fibroids and polyps in premenopausal women. This is particularly important if a woman's primary symptom is heavy menstrual bleeding, since even small submucosal fibroids can be the culprit. The saline-infusion sonogram (SIS) (also known as a sonohysterogram) is the most frequently used technique. This test involves ultrasound but places sterile saltwater (saline) inside the endometrial cavity to expand the uterine cavity (like blowing up a balloon) and allows the inside of the endometrial cavity to be seen (plate 1).[1,2]

A transvaginal ultrasound is usually done first because in some cases submucosal fibroids can be seen without saline infusion. Then a speculum is placed in the vagina to see the cervix just like when a Pap smear is done. The cervix is cleaned with an iodine or soapy solution to decrease the risk of infection and then a small catheter (tube) is passed through the cervix and into the uterus. Some catheters have a small balloon at the tip that is filled with fluid to keep the catheter from slipping out of the cervix. The speculum is removed, and with the catheter in place, the vaginal probe ultrasound can be inserted again to monitor the saline infusion.

Ultrasound pictures are taken as the saline flows into the endometrial cavity. At the end of the procedure, the balloon can be deflated so the area near the cervix can be clearly seen.

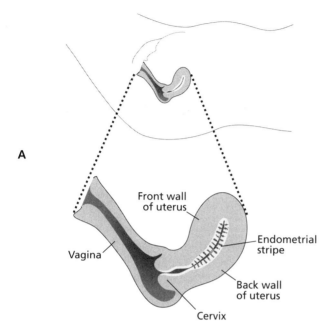

A

Front wall
of uterus

Endometrial
stripe

Vagina

Back wall
of uterus

Cervix

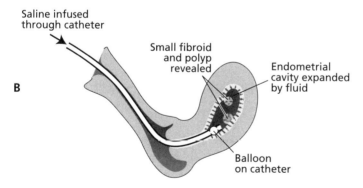

Saline infused
through catheter

Small fibroid
and polyp
revealed

Endometrial
cavity expanded
by fluid

B

Balloon
on catheter

Figure 6.1. In its natural state (6.1A), the endometrial cavity (the inside of the uterus) is collapsed so that the endometrium in the front of the uterus touches the endometrium in the back. When viewed by ultrasound, the two layers of endometrium together are termed the endometrial stripe. In trying to assess the thickness of the endometrial stripe, ultrasonographers measure it from the base of one side to the base of the other. Small fibroids or polyps can sometimes hide in this space. By injecting fluid into the cavity during a saline-infusion sonogram (6.1B), these small lesions can be better seen. However, the physician must carefully look at the images because most catheters have a small balloon near their tip to keep them from falling out of the uterus during the procedure. The balloon can look at first glance like a small fibroid.

Having the catheter placed and the uterus distended can be painful, but for most women, taking over-the-counter medication such as ibuprofen about an hour before the test gives sufficient pain relief. For women with a relatively normal sized uterus the procedure is easily performed. However, for women with large fibroids, two particular problems can arise. First, if the fibroid is in the cervix or near the entrance of the uterus, inserting the catheter can be difficult (or even impossible, though this is rare). Second, if the fibroids are large, the pressure of the saline going into the endometrial cavity may not be enough to open up the cavity. In some instances the cavity seems normal, but really the view is limited, and a big fibroid may be hiding in the top of the cavity.

There are two other tests that can be used to examine the inside of the uterus. Office hysteroscopy involves placing an endoscope inside the uterus to see any lesions directly. The procedure typically uses saline to open up the uterus. The hysteroscopy is usually viewed with a camera and video monitor so both the doctor and the woman can see any lesions. It is more expensive and difficult to perform than a saline-infusion sonogram, but some surgeons prefer this method because they believe it shows more clearly whether the lesions inside the uterus are polyps or submucosal fibroids (plate 2).[3]

Many office hysteroscopy systems use flexible hysteroscopes. Flexible hysteroscopes bend in many different directions, and the end will curl up if pushed against a hard surface. This makes them safer to use than a rigid hysteroscope, which is basically a long metal tube. One of the major risks of hysteroscopy (or any procedure in which something is placed inside the uterus) is uterine perforation, or poking a hole in the uterus. A flexible tube that bends is less likely to go through the uterine wall than a straight, solid tube.

A hysterosalpingogram (HSG) can also be performed. The Greek root of the word tells why this test is sometimes used: *hystero* is uterus, *salpingo* is fallopian tubes, and *gram* is picture. Thus, in this test information is gained about a woman's fallopian tubes in addition to the uterus. When fertility is a goal, an HSG can simultaneously provide information regarding the inside of the uterus and information about possible fallopian tube blockage, a major barrier to pregnancy (plate 3). A few women get pregnant following an HSG. The old theory for these pregnancies was that the dye pushed any sludge through the tubes to open them; a few studies have suggested that the dye used affects some elements of the immune system in a way that could possibly promote pregnancy.

An HSG is generally conceded to be the most uncomfortable ambulatory (outpatient) gynecologic procedure. Women need to take nonsteroidal anti-inflammatory drugs before the procedure; many physicians also place local anesthesia around the cervix to minimize the pain. In addition, HSGs use X-ray guidance and therefore are typically done during the time between the end of a woman's period and ovulation to eliminate the possibility of exposing a very early pregnancy to X-rays. Because an HSG exposes the woman and her ovaries to low doses of radiation, it is usually performed only in women actively trying for pregnancy.

An HSG can be performed several ways, some of which include placing a balloon inside the uterus, just like during a saline-infusion sonogram. Although this is fine for women without fibroids, when only looking at the tubes is important, it can be difficult to differentiate the balloon from a submucosal fibroid. Other ways of performing an HSG involve attaching a device to the outside of the cervix and releasing dye into the cervix, where it can flow into the uterus and tubes. Your doctor should be familiar with the facility where the HSG is done (or perform it him- or herself) to know whether it will provide an adequate evaluation of the inside of the uterus.

Magnetic resonance imaging (MRI) is a test that can provide more precise definition of the uterus (plate 4). It is rarely used as a first test, but it does provide additional information. The MRI machine is a giant doughnut-shaped machine; the patient is on a movable bed inside the doughnut, and the doughnut is a giant magnet. There is no X-ray exposure with MRI, but there is a strong magnetic field, which means that metal objects cannot be taken into or worn inside the device. Jewelry (especially body piercing, which many women forget to mention) needs to be removed before the procedure. People with most electronic implants like pacemakers or defibrillators cannot safely have an MRI; luckily these devices are rare in women with fibroids. The opening in the doughnut is relatively small, and many people experience claustrophobia inside the machine. Wearing an eye mask helps some women. Women weighing more than 250 pounds often cannot fit inside the doughnut for imaging of the abdomen and pelvis. The machine is noisy, too, so most facilities offer earplugs. MRI

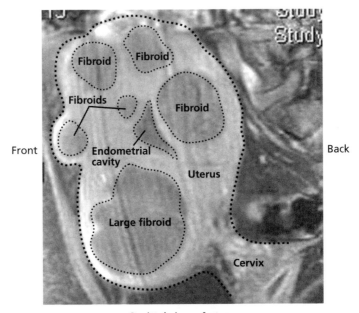

Sagittal view of uterus

Figure 6.2. A T1 weighted MRI image of the uterus after gadolinium has been administered. The uterus and the cervix appear white, indicating that there is good blood flow and the gadolinium has entered that area. There is no blood flow to the crescent-shaped endometrial cavity (center), and none of the six visible fibroids have blood flow. This is because this patient has undergone uterine artery embolization and the blood flow has been cut off.

generally takes an hour to perform and is significantly more expensive than ultrasound.

Often an intravenous catheter (IV) is placed in a hand or arm vein before starting the MRI so that a contrast agent called gadolinium can be used at the end of the procedure. Gadolinium goes through the blood circulation and shows which areas of the uterus or fibroids (or both) do not have good blood flow (fig. 6.2).

MRI more clearly delineates the number of fibroids and their position within the uterus than does ultrasound and can be useful in revealing different diseases.[4] It can differentiate fibroids from another disease process called adenomyosis, which is more difficult to treat (see Chapter 19), and it can give clues about whether the uterine mass is not a typical fibroid but instead a sarcoma or cancer (see Chapter

21).[4] MRI with gadolinium can also assess whether the blood flow has been cut off to the fibroid so that the tissue is dead (degenerated fibroid). All these situations are relatively rare, and therefore the additional cost of an MRI is usually justified only when trying to identify a certain type of fibroid before proceeding with a minimally invasive technique that works only with that type of fibroid. An MRI is clearly less costly than the wrong surgical procedure.

One of the reasons MRI is able to give us more information about many body structures, including the uterus, is that we can take many different sets of pictures within the same study by changing the settings of the MRI scanner. The process is similar to using your camera to take the same picture in black and white and in color. Some features of the image would be seen most clearly in color, while others might be highlighted by the contrast between black and white. With regular X-rays and ultrasounds, tissue density is used to distinguish between two structures. MRI provides extra ways of imaging tissue, which helps us distinguish between things of similar density as well as things of different density.

The two major types of MRI imaging sequences are termed *T1 weighted images* and *T2 weighted images*, or T1 and T2 for short. Instead of measuring density, MRI determines how molecules in tissue respond to the high magnetic field. Fibroids and normal myometrium are best distinguished on T2 images. Most fibroids appear darker than normal myometrium on T2 images (and are thus sometimes called black fibroids). Fluid appears white on these images, so the urine in the bladder and the little bit of fluid in the endometrial cavity appear white on T2 images.

Another advantage of MRI is that magnetic resonance images can predict the outcome of some therapies, particularly uterine artery embolization (UAE) and focused ultrasound surgery (FUS). Therefore MRI can help physicians identify good candidates for minimally invasive therapies based on characteristics other than size and location of fibroids. Some patterns may also be recognizable from ultrasound or other imaging modalities, as well, but they have not yet been categorized and correlated with treatment outcome, as has been done with MRI.

Three-dimensional ultrasound (3D-US) is a new imaging modality that appears to hold promise for the diagnosis of uterine fibroids.[5,6] It employs regular ultrasound technology but takes a sweep of 360 degrees to get a complete picture of the uterus (plate 5). This allows the physician to reconstruct multiple images of the uterus to get a more complete picture of the relationship between structures. It can also be used with SIS. Studies will likely need to be performed to determine how to best use this technology for the diagnosis of fibroids.

Computed tomography (CT scan) usually isn't of great use for the diagnosis of uterine fibroids. However, since contrast agents can be placed in the bowel for a CT scan, on the rare occasions when there is a mass in the pelvis and it is not clear whether the mass is in the bowel or the uterus, this test can be helpful (fig. 6.3). A CT scan does have a significant amount of X-ray exposure, which is a major disadvantage of this imaging modality. A CT also involves a doughnut-like machine and can thus have some of the same confinement limitations that MRI has.

Understanding the orientation of the images is key with imaging. The terms *sagittal, axial,* and *coronal* are used to describe the plane of the image in three dimensions in all types of imaging. Although this terminology is used for ultrasound, it is best understood while looking at images produced by an MRI so that all the structures can be seen. These terms can refer to images of the head or chest, but for the purpose of this book, I will describe pelvic images.

A sagittal scan provides a view of a person as though she were standing sideways; the multiple pictures produced by the scan capture sections of the body from one hip to the other. In these images, your belly is typically on the left side and your back on the right. The sacrum and coccyx (spine and tailbone), for instance, can be seen on the right in images from the middle of the body. The images provided by a sagittal scan give you the best understanding of the relationship of the uterus to the bowel and bladder. They also can give you a view of the endometrial cavity from the top of the fundus down to the cervix if fibroids are not pushing the cavity into a different plane.

An axial scan provides a view of the person lying on her back (which is normally the position a person is in while in the machine), and the images move from the head to the feet. The belly is at the top of the picture and the spine, and the buttocks are at the bottom. Because the viewer is at the foot looking up, the right side of the body

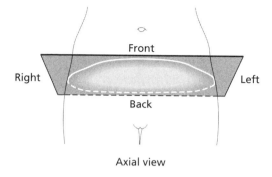

Front

Right

Left

Back

Axial view

Front

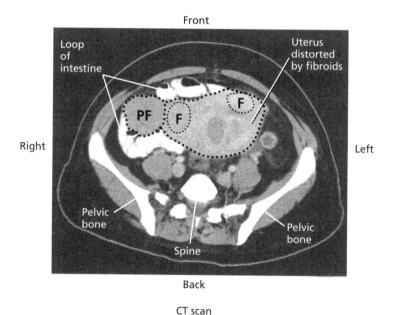

Loop of intestine

Uterus distorted by fibroids

PF

F

F

Right

Left

Pelvic bone

Pelvic bone

Spine

Back

CT scan

Figure 6.3. Computed tomography (CT) scans are rarely used for the assessment of fibroids. They are chiefly useful for being able to tell the difference between a pedunculated fibroid and a mass arising from the bowel. This axial image is best viewed by imagining a woman lying on her back and seeing the image as a cross section through the pelvis. The bones all appear white, and the two sides of the pelvis are easily seen, as is the spine. The bowel also appears white because contrast dye has been placed inside the bowel. The fibroid uterus takes up the majority of the image (two fibroids are labeled with an "F"). The endometrial cavity appears slightly lighter in color. The pedunculated fibroid (labeled "PF") on the far left side of the picture shows bowel surrounding it.

is on the left side of the image. An axial scan can provide a good view for looking at the relationship of the ovaries to the uterus.

A coronal scan provides a view of the person as though she were standing and facing you, and images go from the anterior abdomen through the back. Again, the right side of the body is on the left side of the image. These images can show the relationship of the fibroid to the muscles of the abdominal wall or the back and the bladder.

Looking at all three orientations of images gives you the best appreciation of the relationship between the fibroid uterus and other body structures. Understanding the orientation can help you view the images more effectively yourself.

All current diagnostic tests involve imaging or seeing fibroids in the uterus. Uterine fibroids cannot be detected by any blood or saliva tests. The fact that our treatments are aimed at intervening only after symptoms are present would not currently make these tests particularly useful. However, if we reach the point where we could prevent fibroids, or intervene early to prevent very small fibroids from growing to symptomatic fibroids, other types of less invasive testing would be much more useful.

Currently, the major reason for detecting early fibroid disease is to prevent anemia from prolonged heavy menstrual bleeding. Most women require iron supplementation because of menses-related blood loss, and it is likely that supplementation is even more important for women with fibroids. For women with a Type 0 or I submucosal fibroid, early detection can be important. Since the risks of the surgery are low, treatment is generally recommended as soon as symptoms start. For most other types of fibroids, early intervention is not useful. Some physicians argue that early intervention should be undertaken to prevent the fibroids from growing bigger and causing more problems—what has been termed *prophylactic myomectomy*. Given the high risk of recurrence and some studies suggesting that recurrence may be higher with smaller fibroids, however, prophylactic myomectomy is not recommended.[7]

For the woman contemplating pregnancy, knowing that she has fibroids can be useful. She should know that seeking medical evaluation if she has difficulty getting pregnant or experiences multiple miscarriages is important. Some women who think they are having trouble getting pregnant are in reality having multiple early miscarriages.

Question 2: Do I need to exclude any other process?

Just as important as identifying fibroids is excluding other processes that are causing symptoms we typically attribute to fibroids. The last thing a physician (or his or her patient) wants to do is perform surgery to remove a fibroid and find out that the symptoms that led to that surgery do not improve or that no fibroid exists. A doctor who carefully listens to your symptoms and excludes other possible causes is more likely to reach the right diagnosis.

Diagnosis is relatively easy in women who have an enlarged uterus. If pregnancy is excluded with a blood or urine test, an ultrasound is usually able to rule out the other major cause, which is an ovarian mass. This is why it is useful to do an imaging study within approximately a year of any intervention for fibroids. I have seen patients who knew that they had fibroids from an ultrasound several years earlier and who assumed, based on their symptoms, that the fibroids were growing. When a new ultrasound was done, we found that the fibroids were stable in size but there was now a new large ovarian cyst. We will also discuss in later chapters rare things that need to be excluded in a small subset of women.

Question 3: What should I do if I am having abnormal bleeding?

There are many reasons for abnormal menstrual bleeding besides fibroids. The first clue is the pattern of bleeding. Fibroids, as we discussed in Chapter 1, typically cause heavy or prolonged menstrual bleeding. Bleeding throughout the month is not typical and indicates that further testing needs to be done to exclude a problem with the endometrium, especially endometrial cancer or precancer (endometrial hyperplasia). These problems can be identified or excluded through an endometrial biopsy performed in the office. During an endometrial biopsy, a small plastic tube the size and flexibility of a pipe cleaner is placed into the uterus through the cervix. In most women this can be done without placing any instruments on the cervix. The woman should take over-the-counter pain medication before coming to the office for the procedure. (Larger plastic and metal tubes can be used for biopsies if active bleeding is taking place, to remove more tissue and stop the bleeding.)

When a woman over 35 years old or weighing more than 250 pounds is having abnormal bleeding, performing an endometrial biopsy is especially important, since these women have an increased risk of hyperplasia. Polyps can also sometimes be diagnosed in this way.

There are other causes of heavy bleeding. Failure to ovulate (release an egg) every month, for example, can result in a heavy period. Reproductive-age women as well as older women may fail to ovulate. A woman who does not ovulate is termed *anovulatory,* and one who frequently fails to ovulate is *oligoovulatory.* When ovulation does not occur, the uterine lining builds up in an abnormal fashion because it is being stimulated to grow by estrogen but not organized to fall off by progesterone. Over time, this lining can become unstable and can, in fact, act like a house of cards; once the level gets to a certain point, the cards can fall in an unpredictable manner, and women have heavy, frequent, and irregular bleeding. Ovulation can be assessed in a number of ways: charting the basal body temperature, using urinary ovulation-predictor kits or equipment, or doing blood tests or an endometrial biopsy at specific times in the menstrual cycle.

Thyroid disease can also lead to heavy menses. The thyroid is a small butterfly-shaped gland in the neck that regulates how the body processes energy. Generally, when the thyroid is underactive, heavy menstrual flow results. Other signs of an underactive thyroid include weight gain and fatigue, symptoms that seem universal in reproductive-age women. Many doctors routinely do a thyroid blood test, typically a thyroid-stimulating hormone (TSH), as an initial part of an evaluation for heavy menstrual periods.

Some women have problems with their blood system (hematologic disorders) that make them more likely to have abnormal bleeding when they have fibroids. Identifying a bleeding disorder in a woman who has fibroids is important for two reasons. First, by treating the bleeding disorder, fibroid treatments may potentially be avoided. Second, women with these blood disorders are at risk for postoperative bleeding complications following any surgical or interventional procedure, including treatment of fibroids. These disorders may cause bleeding from procedures ranging from tooth extractions to childbirth. Many of these disorders have a genetic basis, so other family members may also be at risk of bleeding, and therefore it may be a good idea to test family members.

Dozens of different proteins and cells are involved in blood clotting, and looking for all of them in every woman is difficult. There appear to be a small number of disorders that are relatively common in reproductive-age women, however, and by asking some simple questions, doctors can help identify women at high risk of having these disorders.

Experts recommend additional testing for bleeding disorders if a woman experiences any of the following:[8]

- Excessive bleeding since her first period (menarche)
- Hemorrhage following childbirth (postpartum hemorrhage)
- Bleeding related to surgery
- Bleeding associated with dental work

Additional testing is also recommended if a woman experiences two or more of these situations:

- Bruising greater than 5 cm (2 inches) once or twice a month
- Nosebleeds (epistaxis) once or twice a month
- Frequent gum bleeding
- Family history of bleeding disorders

The most common bleeding disorder associated with abnormally heavy menstrual bleeding is Von Willebrand disease (VWD). Although VWD is found in 1–2 percent of all individuals, approximately 10 percent of women with heavy periods have it.[9]

Other, less common causes of abnormal menstrual bleeding include infection of the uterus, medical diseases such as liver disease, and complications related to a previous pregnancy. Tests for these problems are generally not done routinely but may be ordered if a woman's particular problems point in the direction of these rarer causes.

CHAPTER 7

When Fibroids Come Back

Surgically we are beginning to treat more and more fibroids in a minimally invasive fashion. Nonetheless, until we deal with the problem of fibroid recurrence, women will need to have repeated procedures. Fibroid recurrence is not like the recurrence of a cancerous tumor. Cells do not leave the primary fibroid and then reappear later in the same place, or in a distant place, in the body. Rather, recurrence most likely represents the continued formation of new fibroids. In other words, we are getting better at dealing with the fibroids that are big enough to see, feel, or image, but we cannot yet stop the formation process. I classify fibroid recurrence into two different categories: subclinical recurrence and clinical recurrence.

Subclinical recurrence involves any fibroid that can be seen, palpated, or imaged but that may not cause any symptoms (termed having *clinical significance*) or lead to treatment. The risk of a subclinical recurrence is very high. The best published information comes from recurrence after an abdominal myomectomy.[1-5] However, it does appear that there are similar recurrence risks after procedures such as laparoscopic myomectomy and hysteroscopic myomectomy.

Traditionally, subclinical recurrence has been assessed by using ultrasound to image the uterus after surgery. It appears that half of all women will have ultrasound-diagnosed fibroids approximately 5 to 10 years after abdominal myomectomy. (Earlier studies tended to give lower results, but as the imaging improved, more and more fibroids were able to be detected in this manner.) The numbers may be even higher if modalities such as magnetic resonance imaging (MRI) or three-dimensional ultrasound (3D-US) are used in the future to look for new fibroids. For subclinical recurrence a more accurate imaging system will produce higher recurrence rates.

From a woman's point of view, however, the most worrisome type of recurrence is one that leads to another procedure. This is the recurrence that I call *clinical recurrence.* The incidence of clinical recurrence also appears to be high. Following abdominal myomectomy, it appears that a woman has a 15–20 percent chance of having a second major procedure within approximately 10 years. A study we performed in 2002 reinforced these numbers; in fact, when we looked at other, less invasive procedures—including uterine artery embolization (UAE) and dilation and curettage (D&C)—we found that up to one-third of women need to have some type of surgical intervention following an abdominal myomectomy.[5] There are similar chances of recurrence following hysteroscopic myomectomy.[6] Recurrence risk will be a very important issue to assess as new treatments are employed.

With the level of recurrence this high, it is important to predict who is at the highest risk of recurrence. Doing so might help some high-risk women decide that a minimally invasive procedure is a less attractive option, or it may reinforce for low-risk women the conclusion that avoiding hysterectomy is, indeed, the best plan. Older studies suggest that both the number of fibroids present at the initial surgery and having a baby following the surgery are helpful in predicting recurrence risk. A study previously indicated that in women with only one fibroid found during abdominal myomectomy, there was an 11 percent risk of a second surgery, whereas in women with multiple fibroids, there was a 26 percent risk. Other studies suggested that having a term pregnancy (a pregnancy resulting in a birth) following a myomectomy decreased the risk of additional surgery. We followed a group of 65 women who had undergone myomectomy to see whether we could assess new risk factors. One of the drawbacks of this study was that these women were not typical fibroid patients. All women were Caucasian and tended to be thinner than the typical woman with fibroids.

Some of the findings from the study were interesting. First, it appeared that the risk of having a second surgery varied inversely with the size of the uterus and the size of the largest fibroid. In other words, the bigger the fibroid, the less likely a woman was to have a second surgery. At first glance, this does not seem right. Bigger fibroids should represent worse disease and increase the risk of second surgery. We considered two potential reasons for this finding. First, since fibroids are always forming, there may be an advantage to waiting longer. The longer you wait, the bigger the fibroids would tend to get and the easier they would be to remove surgically. It is much easier to find a walnut and remove it than to find a pea. Second, work being done in genetics suggests that bigger fibroids have different chromosome rearrangements.[7] Thus, it may be that bigger fibroids represent a less aggressive kind of fibroid with a particular chromosome pattern and decreased recurrence due to this difference. Studies in a second population showed just the opposite finding, however, and thus larger studies in different populations are required.[8]

We also found that having less weight gain since age 18 decreased the risk of a second surgery. A woman who had gained more than 30 pounds since age 18 had almost a fourfold increased risk of needing a second surgery. There are a number of links between weight and fibroids, as I discussed previously. Gaining weight may represent a hormonal environment that increases recurrence. Again, some of the information from genetics suggests that some of the genes that control body fat may also be important genes in a subtype of uterine fibroids.[9,10]

Finally, we also found some new information: women with a history of endometriosis were more likely to have a second surgery. Although this finding may merely mean that women with fibroids and endometriosis have two reasons to have a second surgery, it could also suggest that there are biological relationships between the two diseases that make the fibroids more aggressive. Heavy periods plus having one or more births led to an increased risk of a second surgery, but this finding may be a confounding factor. It may be that having children does not result in worse fibroids but makes having a second surgery, and potentially a hysterectomy, a less important obstacle.

We clearly need to know more about risk factors for recurrence, particularly in populations of African American women. In addition, it would be useful to know whether hormonal treatment prior to surgery (or other perioperative variables) increases or decreases the risk of recurrence. Evidence regarding the risk of recurrence in women using preoperative gonadotropin-releasing hormone (GnRH) ago-nists, for example, has been mixed, with conflicting results.

The long-term goal, of course, is to decrease the risk of recur-rence. Decreasing this risk may be accomplished in a number of dif-ferent ways: by using medications, by timing the surgery in particu-lar ways, or by proceeding with specific types of procedures. Discovering which approach works best for individual women and for specific types of fibroids is a critically important research goal for the future.

PART II

Surgical Treatment

CHAPTER 8

Surgery Inside the Uterus: Hysteroscopic Myomectomy, Endometrial Ablation, and Vaginal Myomectomy

For some women, hormonal therapy such as birth control pills or progestins can be useful in controlling heavy menstrual periods (menorrhagia). It is not clear whether this treatment truly improves fibroid-related menorrhagia or just treats women who have both fibroids and problems with irregular ovulation or other problems that respond to hormones. We do know that if the symptoms do not significantly improve with the first several cycles, it is unlikely that changing brands of medication will be useful, and moving toward a surgical solution is a better step.

Hysteroscopic Myomectomy

If hormonal therapy does not control a woman's symptoms, then it is important to identify whether there is a submucosal fibroid that can be removed (resected) hysteroscopically. Transvaginal ultrasound, sonohysterogram, hysterosalpingogram (HSG), or diagnostic hysteroscopy can generally be used to diagnose a submucosal fibroid. In the European Society of Hysteroscopy classification, these fibroids that can be treated with a hysteroscope would be Type 0 or Type I fibroids (see Chapter 2).

I described diagnostic hysteroscopy in Chapter 6. But hysteroscopy can also be used for treatment purposes. Although several treatments can be accomplished inside the uterus, hysteroscopic myomectomy is the most important and probably the most underused. A hysteroscopic myomectomy removes a Type 0 or Type I submucosal uterine fibroid by breaking it into pieces and removing it through the cervix (plate 6).

Removal of a submucosal fibroid by hysteroscopic resection has several advantages:

- It is minimally invasive and can be done as an outpatient procedure.
- It has a short recovery time, sometimes as short as 1 or 2 days and usually less than a week.
- A variety of anesthesia choices may be available for this surgery, depending on the institution.
- It appears to be safe for future pregnancies; therefore, it is ideal for young women who want to have children in the future.
- It allows early intervention (small submucosal fibroids are easier to resect than larger ones).

The size of a submucosal fibroid makes a critical difference in whether it can be removed using hysteroscopic surgery. How large a fibroid can be removed depends to some extent on the equipment available and the experience of the surgeon. A rule of thumb is that fibroids less than 3 cm in size can be removed hysteroscopically by most surgeons who do operative hysteroscopy; hysteroscopically resecting fibroids in the range of 3–5 cm is feasible for an expert hysteroscopist. Medications, primarily gonadotropin-releasing hormone (GnRH) agonists (see Chapter 15), can sometimes be used to shrink larger fibroids so they can be resected in this manner. Generally hysteroscopic myomectomy is not recommended for Type II fibroids.[1]

Several instruments can be used to resect a fibroid. The traditional device is the resectoscope, a rigid scope originally used for prostate surgery and then adapted for gynecologic use. The size of hysteroscopes used in the operating room is larger than ones used in the office because they need to accommodate use of operative equipment. This instrument typically uses a wire loop electrode, which allows pieces to be cut out of the fibroid and removed. Resectoscopes traditionally use a non-salt-containing solution, such as sorbitol or glycine, to fill the uterus. (Because a salt solution would dissipate the electrical current, the resectoscope would not be able to work properly.) A major problem with these fluids is that they can be absorbed into the body. The uterus can act like a sponge and directly take the fluid into the bloodstream, or fluid can go out through the fallopian tubes and more slowly be absorbed into the bloodstream through the abdominal cavity. This absorption of fluid is a problem because it can change the body-salt composition or electrolyte balance. A runner needs to replace fluid with Gatorade and not water because major shifts in electrolytes can cause significant problems and even, rarely, death.[2,3] The same principle applies here.

Prevention is usually the first step in minimizing the complications with these fluids. Most institutions have fluid-monitoring devices and prearranged stop points. Even if this is not the case and a significant imbalance develops, prompt recognition and treatment with a change in intravenous fluids and diuretics (drugs that cause the body to increase excretion of fluids) can remedy this problem.

Newer generations of hysteroscopes have been designed that work with salt-containing solution. Examples include resectoscopes that work with saline and a new system that uses mechanical resection.[4] The latter device also removes the pieces resected from the uterus with suction to minimize the amount of operating time required. Because it is a simpler system, it may be also easier to use than traditional devices.

Endometrial Ablation

A second strategy for controlling fibroid-related bleeding is to ignore the fibroids in the uterus but to destroy the uterine lining. If there is no uterine lining, there is nothing to bleed—even in the presence of fibroids. The procedure for destroying the uterine lining in a minimally invasive way is called an *endometrial ablation*.

Unfortunately, endometrial ablation devices are typically designed for and tested on women who do not have uterine fibroids. Even though these devices are widely used to treat women with fibroid-related bleeding, their primary use is for heavy menstrual bleeding in women who have a structurally normal uterus. Therefore, two issues need to be addressed before an endometrial ablation can be performed. First, a thorough assessment of the endometrial cavity needs to be done to see whether a submucosal fibroid is present. If one is found, an endometrial ablation can be performed in conjunction with a hysteroscopic myomectomy. Second, some devices for endometrial ablation can accommodate an irregular cavity, but others cannot. Table 8.1 lists many devices for endometrial ablation and their advantages and disadvantages.

Following endometrial ablation, many women who begin with a *normal* uterine cavity have no menstrual bleeding (amenorrhea). But amenorrhea appears to be very rare in women with fibroids who undergo endometrial ablation. My clinical impression is that nearly all women having the procedure have the same magnitude of improvement but, because they don't begin at the same place, they don't reach the same endpoint. If you are starting with 8 days of very heavy bleeding, getting to 4 days of normal bleeding is the same degree of improvement as starting at 4 days of moderate bleeding and getting to no menstrual bleeding.

Endometrial ablation should not be considered an option for women who desire future fertility, since the goal of ablation is to destroy the entire endometrium, including the basalis layer, so that the normal lining does not grow back (as discussed in Chapter 2, it is the basalis layer that directs the regeneration of endometrial tissue). The removal of the basalis is the reason that endometrial ablation works better to control bleeding than the older procedure of dilatation and curettage (D&C), in which only the functionalis layer of the endometrium is removed. In fact, in the age of hysteroscopy and biopsy, some doctors have questioned whether the D&C is an outmoded procedure.[5]

Women nonetheless still need to use birth control after an ablation. Destroying the lining does not prevent the egg and the sperm from joining and producing a pregnancy; it only produces a less optimal environment for the pregnancy to grow inside the uterus. Pregnancies outside the uterus can and do occur, including tubal and cervical pregnancies. Even intrauterine pregnancies have occurred after endometrial ablation, though these have been rare.

You can never assume, however, that the endometrium is 100 percent destroyed in an endometrial ablation. Intrauterine pregnancies

Table 8.1. Approaches to Endometrial Ablation

Device	Mechanism	Advantages	Disadvantages
Resectoscope	Can physically remove endometrium with loop or destroy by contact using roller bar or roller ball	Can accommodate any size cavity. Same equipment for hysteroscopic myomectomy. Provides specimen for pathology.	Requires advanced surgical skills. Best results with thin endometrium. Medical pretreatment often required.
Thermal balloon (Thermachoice, Cavaterm)	Hot water contained in a balloon leads to thermal destruction of endometrium	Easy to use	Limited size and shape of cavities able to be treated. Ablation based on time, so variations in endometrium are limiting.
Microwave (MEA)	Sweep of wand	Women with leiomyomas included in original trials	Moving wand more operator-dependent. Requires ultrasound measurement of uterine wall thickness prior to procedure.
Bipolar mesh (Novasure)	Bipolar electrode mesh conforms to cavity and radio frequency (RF) energy vaporizes and coagulates endometrium. Suction removes steam and tissue as ablation performed.	Easy to use. Checks for intact cavity prior to ablation. Impedence-regulated device can accommodate a variety of endometrial thicknesses.Conforms to irregular cavities.	Restricted to small cavities
Hydrotherm ablation	Free-flowing hot water with hysteroscopic visualization	Can accommodate any size cavity. Real-time visualization.	Potential for vaginal burns

have occurred following endometrial ablation because the endometrium wasn't completely destroyed.

Likewise, if abnormal patterns of bleeding occur at any time following endometrial ablation, an endometrial biopsy needs to be performed to rule out endometrial cancer. People were initially concerned that, following endometrial ablation, the inside walls of the uterus would stick together and, if cancer developed, it could be hidden inside the uterus, but this does not seem to be the case. Just like women with no prior surgery, women with endometrial cancer who have had an endometrial ablation have abnormal uterine bleeding. However, women who are obese or who do not ovulate regularly and are therefore at risk of endometrial hyperplasia may not be optimal candidates for ablation and should be counseled about this risk prior to the ablation.

An intrauterine device (IUD) containing a progestin (Mirena is the brand name of the device, and levonorgestrel is the progestin it contains) is also used to produce what some people have termed a reversible medical endometrial ablation.[6,7] Studies have documented that, although in general the decrease in blood loss achieved with surgical ablation is greater, both approaches give women significant relief from bleeding problems. For the woman who also needs contraception or who is not certain about her plans for future pregnancy, the IUD can be a better option. Other, nonmedicated IUDs don't seem to have the same benefit and can lead to heavier periods. Most authorities recommend using an IUD only when the woman is in a mutually monogamous relationship (neither she nor her partner has any other sexual partners) to avoid the risk of pelvic inflammatory disease.

Vaginal Myomectomy

Rarely, a fibroid that starts out as a submucosal fibroid extrudes itself through the cervix and into the vagina. When the doctor places a speculum in the vagina, he or she observes a fibroid that appears to be sitting there and is often the size of a golf ball. The extrusion is often preceded by what women describe as laborlike pain. This makes sense, since much of labor involves dilating, or gradually opening, the cervix, and this is what is literally happening as the fibroid works its way out. Women also tend to report intermittent gushing-type bleeding with this process. Some women I have seen have experienced the bleeding symptoms but not the laborlike pain. These fibroids that tend to be located in the cervix before moving into the vagina seem to be very difficult to see by most imaging techniques.

Physicians are not used to looking for a dilated cervix in these circumstances. I have seen ultrasound and HSGs in which this situation was missed as well as hysteroscopies in which a large fibroid was not seen. If the physician is not specifically looking for this kind of fibroid, he or she will often not see it.

Once the fibroid has popped through the cervix and is in the vagina, however, physicians act to remove it quickly to prevent ascending infection. (With the cervix held open by the fibroid, the bacteria that fill the vagina may more easily go up, or ascend, into the uterus and fallopian tubes.)

What makes removing these vaginal fibroids difficult is controlling the blood loss. They often have very thick stalks with large blood vessels. Getting around the fibroid to clamp, tie, or cauterize the stalk is the challenging part. Because most gynecologists have never seen a prolapsed submucosal fibroid, the situation poses a challenge. Even in my specialty fibroid practice, I see only about one a year.

CHAPTER 9

Laparoscopic Myomectomy and Myolysis

Laparoscopic myomectomy and myolysis are two more recent approaches to fibroids that offer a minimally invasive option for some women who previously would have needed major abdominal surgery. Both of these treatments deal best with subserosal fibroids (ones located closer to the outer surface of the uterus). A laparoscopic myomectomy removes the fibroid from the uterus and then repairs the normal myometrium by sewing (suturing) it back together.[1] Myolysis uses a laser fiber or needles that deliver an electric current to destroy the fibroid in the uterus.[2] In either procedure fibroids may recur, since the procedures target fibroids that are present but do not stop the process that is producing fibroids. In addition, one or two subserosal fibroids may be treated with this approach and others present at the time of surgery not treated.

Laparoscopic myomectomy was first used, and is still most widely used, for fibroids that are pedunculated, or on a stalk. For these fibroids, the removal is relatively easy, since the stalk can often be grasped, tied, or burned to control blood loss. The more challenging issue has been removing a large fibroid through a small incision.

Laparoscopic myomectomy is monitored with a laparoscope (similar to a telescope) that is inserted through a small incision at the belly button, just like in a laparoscopic tubal ligation ("having your tubes tied"). Instruments inserted into one or two smaller incisions lower on the abdominal wall are used to grasp the fibroid and uterus.

Cautery or other cutting instruments separate the fibroid from the normal myometrium. The fibroid can then be removed (fig. 9.1).

One of the earliest ways of removing the fibroid was to make an incision into the vagina (colpotomy) and remove the fibroid through that opening.[3] This was a shorter procedure than trying to cut the fibroid into little pieces and remove them through the abdominal incisions. The introduction of electric morcellators, by which the fibroid can be rapidly processed into little pieces, was a major step forward. This advance made it possible to remove large fibroids in a minimally invasive fashion.

Surgeons with advanced skills can remove deeper or even multiple fibroids in this way. One issue with deeper fibroids is that it's more difficult to completely separate them from the underlying myometrium. Another is that the uterus must also be sutured, or stitched, back together.

The difference between regular suturing and laparoscopic suturing is similar to that between walking and walking on stilts. The principles of laparoscopic suturing are the same as those of regular suturing, but a significant amount of practice is required to carry out the moves with the same precision and grace.

The difficulty of laparoscopic suturing is one of the primary reasons some gynecologists have started to explore the possibility of using a surgical robot to perform laparoscopic myomectomy.[4] In robotic myomectomy, the surgeon sits at a console, which can be in the operating room or can be thousands of miles away. From this console, the surgeon controls the robot, which duplicates the surgeon's hand movements. With current robots, the surgeon can view the surgery in three dimensions. Not only is the view more like performing an open surgery than looking through a scope, but the robot allows the surgeon to use all the subtle, fine motions his or her hand can make that are impossible to perform with the stiltlike laparoscopic instruments. Finally, the console allows the surgeon to sit comfortably rather than standing in a specific position to perform the laparoscopy, resulting in less strain and more efficiency. The robotic arm controlled by the surgeon does require time to set up at the beginning of the case and a second surgeon to assist with conventional instruments.

For laparoscopic myomectomies, even with a skilled surgeon, sometimes the time under anesthesia can be significantly longer than for an open procedure. Although incisions are minimized and bleed-

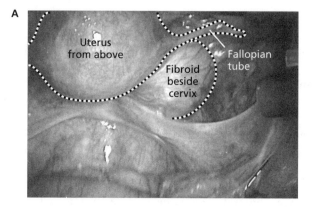

Figure 9.1A. A fibroid is in the right broad ligament (out beside the cervix). The uterus is pushed to the left upper portion of the image. In this image you can also see the thin, sheetlike peritoneum (which becomes the serosa over the uterus) covering all the pelvic contents.

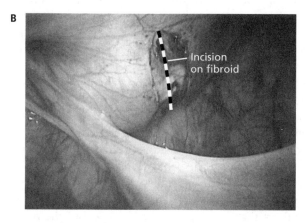

Figure 9.1B. A small incision is made through the peritoneum and down to the level of the fibroid.

ing may be minimized, a significantly longer procedure can be a disadvantage. Women should discuss with their surgeons typical times and outcomes for this procedure.

Finally, some uteruses are too large to allow fibroids to be removed laparoscopically. If the uterus rises above the belly button, a laparoscope placed in this region cannot easily monitor the procedure.

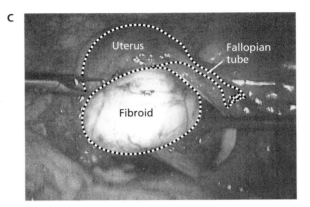

Figure 9.1C. The fibroid has almost been removed. The instrument in the upper left corner grasps the fibroid and allows it to be moved around, while the instrument on the right separates the fibroid from the underlying tissue. The right fallopian tube is also easily viewed.

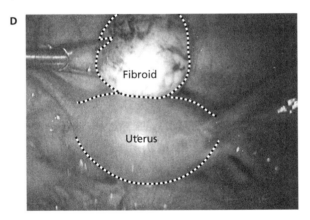

Figure 9.1D. The fibroid is completely removed and is placed in front of the uterus prior to removal. A device called a morcellator allows the fibroid to be taken out in pieces, to avoid making a large incision.

Some physicians do place the laparoscope higher in the abdomen, but eventually the amount of space that is available for operating becomes limited.

Myolysis does not require as much surgical skill as laparoscopic myomectomy. Generally, the probes (or needles) need to be inserted into the fibroid, but the uterus usually does not need to be sutured.

Multiple punctures are required to treat even a small fibroid, and the serosal layer of the uterus is damaged by this technique, which may result in more scarring following surgery. The scarring can cause pain or problems for women trying for pregnancy.

The major controversy over laparoscopic myomectomy and my-olysis has involved the group of women who want to have a future pregnancy, since when these procedures were relatively new, there were several reports of women who experienced uterine rupture at approximately 7 to 8 months of pregnancy.[5-9] Uterine rupture occurs when the uterine wall gives way before labor. It can be a medical emergency for both the mother and the baby. In some of the cases of rupture after these procedures, both mother and baby did well after an emergency cesarean section, but some babies died as a result of the uterine rupture.

Significant controversy continues over this issue in the medical literature. Some authorities argue that inadequate surgical skill led to these early complications. While this concern may have some validity, there is also evidence that even superficial disruption of the serosal uterine lining may sometimes lead to uterine rupture.[8] Although some surgeons have argued that removing the fibroid laparoscopically but making a bigger incision to repair the uterus directly is the solution, uterine ruptures have also occurred with this approach.[8]

Large studies of a significant number of women are beginning to be published which suggest that the rates of uterine rupture are less than 1 in 100 to 1 in several hundred.[10,11] However, since uterine rupture is such a serious complication for both mother and baby, even a rate of rupture of 1 in several thousand may not be acceptable. Given the complexity of the process, best results will likely occur with surgeons who perform a high volume of these specialized procedures. Women who desire future fertility should discuss the issue of uterine rupture with their surgeon before undergoing a laparoscopic myomectomy.

CHAPTER 10

Abdominal Myomectomy

Abdominal myomectomy is a major surgical procedure in which uterine fibroids are removed from the uterus and the uterus is then repaired (fig. 10.1). This procedure is advantageous for women with symptomatic fibroids that are either too large or too numerous to be removed using laparoscopic myomectomy. It is also the current treatment of choice for most women who are actively trying for pregnancy. A problem with this procedure, as with all surgical procedures used to remove fibroids, is that there is a high risk of recurrent fibroids. Surgical procedures can remove whatever fibroids are present at a particular time, but they do not stop the process of fibroid formation, and new ones may develop.

Some studies have suggested that myomectomy has a greater incidence of surgical *morbidity* (bad side effects or complications but not death—which is termed *mortality*) than hysterectomy, but most studies suggest that these two procedures are similar with regard to such problems.[1-3] Still, an abdominal myomectomy does violate many of the principles of surgical therapy; therefore, when performed by less experienced surgeons, it may be a riskier procedure. It is important, then, to choose a surgeon with significant experience.

Surgical procedures are usually begun by controlling the major blood vessels, but this cannot be done in a myomectomy because the procedure is designed to save the uterus, and therefore the major blood supply cannot be cut off. A number of strategies have evolved to limit blood loss at the time of surgery. Women contemplating abdominal

Figure 10.1A. The uterus before the surgery begins. A 6-inch ruler is on the left, and the front of the uterus is on this side. The fallopian tube and ovary are at the bottom of the picture, and most of the fibroid is protruding from the backside of the uterus.

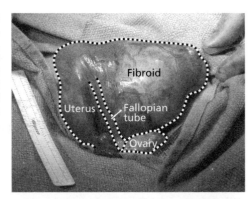

Figure 10.1B. The fibroid, after it has been removed.

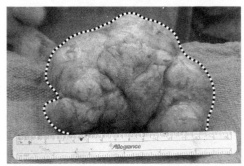

Figure 10.1C. The normal uterus from the front with both fallopian tubes and ovaries. A seam closed the back of the uterus where the fibroid was removed.

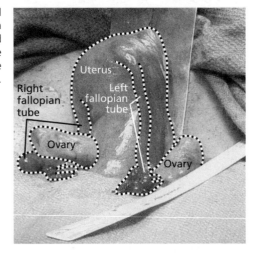

Figure 10.1. An abdominal myomectomy removes the fibroids and repairs or reconstructs the uterus.

myomectomy should be aware of the options (described below) and discuss them with their surgeon. Not all surgical procedures have to be identical, but being aware of all the options is important.

Minimizing Blood Loss

To prevent excessive blood loss or the consequences of this kind of blood loss, the following five options should be considered:

1. Maximize preoperative blood count. Women contemplating surgery for uterine fibroids should be taking iron and vitamins to increase their hematocrit (the percentage of red blood cells) prior to surgery. The degree to which a woman has anemia before the procedure dictates the amount of iron that may be necessary. Given that many women with fibroids are chronically anemic due to menstrual blood loss, iron intake is especially important. Many physicians recommend iron for women who are anemic as a result of having fibroids, but they neglect to recommend multivitamins. Many vitamins are necessary to make new red blood cells, and thus the combination is important.

    This is an approach most women should use. It is relatively inexpensive and easy to do. The major limiting factor is that taking iron supplements commonly causes constipation. This can be particularly annoying when the fibroids are also pressing on the bowel and contributing to constipation as well. There are, however, many different formulations of iron including pills and liquids, pills coupled with stool softeners, and slow-release formulations. If you have significant constipation, it is worth working with your doctor and your pharmacist to find a better iron supplement for you.

2. If iron and vitamins alone do not resolve the anemia, there are several alternative strategies for raising the blood count. The most common is the use of drugs called gonadotropin-releasing hormone (GnRH) agonists (Lupron, Zoladex, and Synarel). These drugs, which work by shutting down the reproductive system at the level of the hypothalamus, are discussed in detail in Chapter 15. They first cause an increase in hormones, called the flare, and then a few weeks later they cause a state commonly called a "medical menopause." The "medical menopause" phase is an advantage

for treating fibroids because it creates menopausal levels of estrogen and progesterone and causes more than 90 percent of women to stop having periods. During the initial, or flare, phase, some women have a very heavy flow that, for women with severe anemia, can be a significant problem.

The "medical menopause" state is associated with hot flashes and bone loss, as is normal menopause. These side effects limit the long-term effectiveness and safety of this approach to resolving anemia, but the Food and Drug Administration (FDA) has approved the use of Lupron in the preoperative management of uterine fibroids when used with iron in preparation for surgery. This is the only FDA-approved medical treatment for uterine fibroids. However, other GnRH agonists should work in a similar fashion. GnRH agonists are the most widely used drugs for inducing amenorrhea (the lack of periods) prior to surgery. Other drugs, such as continuous birth control pills, progesterone, synthetic progestins, and danazol (synthetic androgen), also may successfully stop menstruation. The GnRH agonists also decrease the size of the uterus, which is not the case with these other drugs and the reason that GnRH agonists are more widely used for preoperative treatment. A smaller uterus can also make surgery easier.

3. Intraoperative blood loss can be limited by specific surgical techniques. The most common are the use of a tourniquet, the injection of a drug called vasopressin into the myometrium, the use of arterial clamps, and the Cell Saver.[4-7] A tourniquet places pressure over the major blood vessels leading to the uterus and thus decreases the blood flow during the operation. Significant surgical skill is needed to place a tourniquet safely, since there are many blood vessels and other vital structures in this area. In addition, certain fibroids arising from the lower uterine segment or the cervix make it difficult to safely place a tourniquet in all cases. The second strategy to limit blood loss is injecting a dilute solution of vasopressin into the myometrium. This causes local blood vessel constriction. Vasopressin is a natural hormone that is made by the pituitary gland. It is used in a very dilute solution over the points where incisions are made for the myomectomy but can cause significant problems if injected into the circulation. Some surgeons place vascular clamps over the ovarian arteries and veins while operating. Finally, instruments such as the Cell Saver can be used

intraoperatively. The Cell Saver allows blood that is normally lost during surgery to be filtered and processed so that the patient's red blood cells can be returned to her. Instead of going through a suction tube and being discarded, the red blood cells are saved and given back through the intravenous (IV) line like a transfusion, but with your own blood.

4. With women who have persistent anemia, sometimes either intravenous iron infusion or erythropoietin can be used to stimulate blood production. Many women with fibroids have an iron deficiency, and some women cannot absorb enough iron from their intestines with liquid iron or iron tablets. Intravenous iron infusion is useful only with women who are very iron-deficient. Intravenous iron can cause serious allergic reactions and needs to be carefully supervised. It is usually done only in a hospital setting. Erythropoietin, on the other hand, is the body's natural hormone for stimulating blood production. It is unnecessary in most women with iron deficiency because the body is already naturally stimulating the production. However, in certain circumstances, such as women who need significant blood replacement but cannot have a blood transfusion because they are Jehovah's Witnesses (for example), erythropoietin can be an option.

5. Finally, the use of autologous blood transfusion can be useful. If you are able to build up your blood count, then several units of your own blood can be extracted and stored for your later use. Donating the units of blood will stimulate additional blood production, and if transfusion is required during surgery, receiving your own blood poses less risk than receiving blood donated from someone else. This option is not available as an emergency strategy; it does not help to give blood on Monday for use during surgery on Wednesday. At least several weeks are needed to build up the blood count to normal following donation of a unit of blood before you can safely have surgery.

Incisions

Abdominal myomectomies require an abdominal incision. The size can range from a "bikini" cut (a very small horizontal incision that can be hidden by a bikini bottom) to a large vertical incision, extending above the belly button. Although surgical skill is a factor in the surgeon's choice of which incision to use, with women who have fibroids a significant factor in making this decision is the size of the uterus. If the fibroids extend way above the belly button and up toward the liver, then trying to remove these fibroids through a bikini incision is impossible, or at least ill advised. Sometimes, however, there are other options.

Just as either a vertical or a horizontal bikini incision can be used to cut into the skin, the deeper layers of the abdominal wall can be approached in different ways, too. Using a short horizontal cut on the outside, for example, does not always mean that the same type of incision has to be used on the inside.

The most common type of incision is a Pfannenstiel. With this incision, the surgeon makes a bikini cut in the skin but does not continue to cut horizontally through the major abdominal muscles (the rectus abdominus); the two sides of the rectus abdominus, or the muscle bellies, are separated in the midline instead. Thus, the deeper layer has a vertical incision, which explains why women with this kind of incision can have postoperative pain near the belly button, far from the incision they see. The rectus muscles limit the amount of room that can be used to operate with a Pfannenstiel incision. The bladder also limits the room at the base of the incision. Generally a Pfannenstiel incision leads to less postoperative pain and better functioning of the abdominal muscles after surgery, but it does not always give the surgeon enough room to deal with all of the fibroids.

A Maylard incision consists of a bikini cut through the skin and a transverse incision in the deeper layers. This means that the rectus muscles are cut crosswise. Because this incision provides more room to work, it can allow a larger uterus to be approached without resorting to a vertical incision. However, a Maylard incision may result in more postoperative discomfort and more difficulty getting the muscles to work normally following surgery.

Traditionally, a vertical incision has been avoided not only because it is cosmetically less attractive but also because of concerns that it will pose more difficulty in healing. Because all the blood vessels that go to the abdominal wall come from near the spine and back and then meet in the midline, at the front of the body, the midline has less blood supply, making it less able to heal. In practice, however, for most women with fibroids who are young and healthy, this does not appear to be a major issue.

Sometimes it is difficult to make a final decision until the day of surgery. In addition to the size of the uterus, the mobility of the uterus (how easily it moves) can be important in deciding which incision is appropriate. Mobility is much easier to assess when a woman has had anesthesia and is not uncomfortable. Rarely, the uterus feels significantly bigger or smaller in the operating room than it did in the office. Having an updated imaging study like an ultrasound significantly decreases the possibility that the uterus will be unexpectedly large or small, but surprises do sometimes happen.

We typically gauge the size of the fibroid uterus by its relationship to the pelvic bones, just as we do for the pregnant uterus. However, with uterine fibroids, there can also be substantial volume behind the uterus and in fact below or behind the cervix, and this volume can be very important in the surgical approach. Without taking this volume into account, the size of the uterus is underestimated.

Likewise, the uterine size will usually be overestimated in a heavier woman, since the surgeon is feeling the size of the uterus with the intervening abdominal wall. If the abdominal wall is 2 inches thick, the uterus will "feel" much bigger than if the wall is a quarter of an inch thick. It is almost like having the same package and putting different amounts of wrapping around it. Keeping these two factors in mind, a skilled surgeon is better able to gauge the correct size of incision needed.

Surgical Complications and How to Minimize Them

To minimize the risk of postoperative infection, most physicians prescribe at least one dose of antibiotics to be given through the IV right before the surgery starts. Some physicians continue antibiotics for their patients for the first 24 hours, as well.

Another concern is the risk of blood clots in the legs (deep venous thrombosis, or DVT). Clots that form in the legs may break off and move toward the lungs (pulmonary embolus, or PE); this is a more serious threat than DVT. There are several strategies for decreasing the risk of DVTs (and thus PEs), including physical compression and injections of blood-thinning agents. Compression devices include elastic stockings and pneumoboots (boots that puff air around the lower legs during the surgery). Blood thinners are typically started prior to the surgery. Both compression devices and blood thinners are continued until the woman is up and walking.

Preventing adhesions (bands of scar tissue that bind two parts of tissue together) is also important following myomectomy and is particularly important for women planning pregnancies. Surgical technique in terms of the types of incisions, the suture used, and the handling of tissue appears to be a factor in the formation of adhesions.

In the past, attempts to minimize adhesions involved instilling various fluids or drugs (or both) into the abdomen following surgery. This approach has largely been replaced by various adhesion barriers placed over the uterine incisions to keep other structures from sticking to the uterus. Although a number of agents have been tested, there is no consensus on the ideal regimen, and just like other myomectomy issues, discussing adhesions and their prevention with your surgeon is useful prior to surgery.

Teachings about abdominal myomectomy also suggest that, for a woman who becomes pregnant after undergoing this procedure, a cesarean section should be required if the myomectomy incision goes all the way through the uterine wall and into the endometrial cavity. Although there is no clear evidence that a cesarean section (also referred to as a C-section) is required, it has long been a practice and has resulted in many healthy pregnancies for both mother and baby. The practice was initially begun because it was well established that having a cesarean section with a vertical uterine incision (a classical C-section) increased the risk of uterine rupture in a subsequent pregnancy. In the initial studies that reported this risk with classical C-section, the risk of uterine rupture with myomectomy was also assessed. The risk of uterine rupture following myomectomy was significantly lower than what was seen following classical C-section.[8] There are many ways in which a myomectomy is a very different procedure than a cesarean section. Nonetheless, C-section after abdominal myomectomy is the usual practice, and few practitioners deviate from this teaching.

Finally, given the high risk of recurrent surgery following abdominal myomectomy, I believe the strategy should be to remove all fibroids that are visible or palpable (able to be felt). Using many of the aforementioned techniques minimizes risks, and there are very few fibroids that are "too dangerous" to remove.

CHAPTER 11

Uterine Artery Embolization

Uterine artery embolization (UAE), also referred to as uterine fibroid embolization (UFE), is a minimally invasive treatment for uterine fibroids (fig. 11.1). (The term *ablation*, as in endometrial ablation, and the term *embolization* sound similar and can be easily confused.) The principle behind embolization treatment is that by temporarily blocking off the blood supply to the uterus, the fibroids are destroyed and the normal myometrium is able to recover.

This embolization technique has been used for many years to treat emergencies of uterine bleeding, including bleeding after childbirth or with certain kinds of abnormal pregnancies. It was first used specifically for uterine fibroids in 1995. The original study by Ravina and associates treated women prior to planned hysterectomy.[1] Because a significant proportion of the women had symptom relief without undergoing surgery, the technique was explored as an alternative to hysterectomy. Because the catheters and embolic agents used for UAE treatment were widely used for the treatment of other diseases, UAE was rapidly incorporated into practice.[2-5] (There was not a "new" device introduced that would have required clinical trials supervised by the U.S. Food and Drug Administration [FDA] before the device could be used.) However, since that time, clinical trials have been conducted, and several embolic agents have received approval from the FDA specifically to treat symptomatic uterine fibroids. (Prior to this time, use for fibroid treatment was what is termed "off-label" use.)

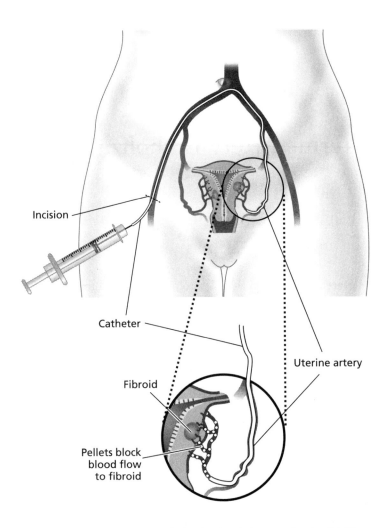

Incision

Catheter

Uterine artery

Fibroid

Pellets block blood flow to fibroid

Figure 11.1. In uterine artery embolization (UAE) the procedure itself is like a cardiac catheterization. A small incision is made where the leg meets the trunk, and a thin, spaghetti-like tube called a catheter is placed in the major blood vessel (artery). Instead of moving the catheter up to the heart and using a balloon at the tip to open up the blood vessel, the catheter is first placed in the opposite uterine artery. Once the catheter is in the correct place, small pellets (like grains of sand) are released, and they flow downstream into the uterus as seen in the circular insert. Catheters small enough to reach individual fibroids are not available, but the size and shape of the particles help to direct them preferentially to the fibroids rather than to normal myometrium. The catheter is then moved back and repositioned, and the second uterine artery (on the side where the catheter is inserted) is embolized in the same way.

The Procedure

As a procedure, embolization is very similar to a cardiac catheterization. UAE takes place in a room with fluoroscopy equipment to take X-ray pictures throughout and have them available on a screen to guide the procedure. An incision less than a half an inch in size is made where the leg meets the trunk. This allows the artery to be identified, and a long skinny tube called a *catheter* is then put into the blood vessel under X-ray guidance. Instead of taking the catheter up to the heart and using a balloon to open up a blood vessel, the catheter is used to go to both the right and left uterine arteries and uses tiny sandlike pellets (embolic agents) to block off the blood supply to the uterus.

The pellets are normally made of polyvinyl alcohol (PVA) or trisacryl gelatin microspheres (TGM) and are designed to stay in the blood vessels permanently. "Dissolving" embolic agents are available, but most of the time fibroid embolization is done with one of the permanent agents. Many women are concerned that the particles will move at some later date and possibly injure another organ. Once they are in the uterine blood vessels, however, this is unlikely. There have been rare complications with pellets going to other places in the pelvis and causing injury to the labia or buttocks, but these complications probably occurred because the pellets were released too early and went down other branches of the major blood vessels in the pelvis and not just the uterine arteries.[6,7] Finding a physician who does a lot of pelvic embolization is essential.

Many people have the impression that the blood supply to a specific fibroid can be targeted, since some academic papers discuss things such as "superspecific UAE." This is not possible, however, and that is why I prefer the older term *UAE* to *UFE*. Uterine artery embolization is a global therapy: it targets the whole uterus, including normal myometrium and endometrium. Two things help optimize placement of the pellets. First, placing the catheter deeply into the uterine artery so that the flow is forward into the uterus is crucial. Second, the size and shape of the embolic agent used determine whether you block the vessel closer to the origin or closer to the fibroid. The smaller and rounder the embolic agents are, the farther they flow. Just as if you were trying to block off the branch of a creek, you are better off using big logs than little branches and better off using logs than beachballs the same size.

The procedure generally takes about an hour. Patients receive local anesthesia, or numbing medication similar to what you get in the dentist's office, for the small incision as well as intravenous medication for relaxation and pain relief during the procedure. The goal is to be awake but relaxed. In most institutions, patients are hospitalized the first night after the procedure. UAE is associated with a high chance of fever and pain postoperatively. This combination of symptoms is commonly referred to as postembolization syndrome.[8,9] The pain of postembolization syndrome can be quite severe and can be like "having a heart attack in your uterus." Heart attack pain is caused when the heart muscle has its blood supply cut off, so it makes sense that cutting off the blood supply to the uterus produces similar pain. Pain medications are provided to minimize the pain, and experiencing significant pain is now rare following UAE.

Most women are discharged from the hospital the next morning, and most women require a narcotic pain medication while at home. Early studies documented that women return to work in 7 to 10 days; more recent studies suggest that many women may return to work after less than a week, with the full range being about 4 to 14 days.

The Results of UAE

Most studies reveal that more than 80 percent of women have a reduction in their fibroid-related bleeding; a similar percentage have a reduction in the symptoms related to the size of their fibroids. Many women erroneously assume that this means that UAE reduces the volume of the uterus by 80 percent. In fact, the average uterine volume reduction is about 30 percent, which is a disappointment for many women. Translating this volume reduction into the expected size of the fibroid following embolization is complex.

One of the major issues is the relationship between diameter and volume (my thanks to my colleague Dr. Mark Emanuel of the Netherlands for reminding me of this issue). The formula for calculating the volume of a sphere is $0.525 \, D^3$, where D is the diameter of the sphere. (Most fibroids are not spherical but are really ellipsoids, more like a baking potato than an orange, with several different diameters.) This formula also works in those cases using $D_1{}^*D_2{}^*D_3$ (representing the diameter in each dimension) instead of D^3.

Table 11.1. Diameter and Volume of the Uterus before and after Uterine Artery Embolization (UAE)

Pre UAE		Post UAE (30% decrease in volume)	
Diameter (cm)	Volume (cm³)	Diameter (cm)	Volume (cm³)
1	0.5	0.8	0.4
2	4.2	1.7	2.9
3	14.2	2.7	9.9
5	65.6	4.4	45.9
10	525.0	8.9	367.0
15	1,814.0	13.4	1,270.0

In table 11.1, the first two columns show the diameter and the volume for several different sizes of spherical fibroids. (Although most fibroids are not spheres, using a single value for all three dimensions makes the concept easier to grasp.) In the last two columns we see the diameter and volume of those same fibroids if the typical 30 percent volume reduction occurs following UAE.

The first thing to note is that the volume rises quickly as the diameter increases. The volume of a 10-cm fibroid is 1,000 times greater than a 1-cm fibroid. Most people erroneously assume that with a 30 percent volume reduction (i.e., the volume is reduced by about a third), the diameter will be decreased by about a third. But that is not the case, and so, instead of the diameter of a 15-cm fibroid shrinking by 5 cm, it shrinks only by 1.6 cm. Thus many women with big fibroids who expect to have a flat stomach following UAE are disappointed with their results.

The other way in which to relieve symptoms is to change the pressure or composition of the mass. Fibroids are typically firm and rubbery. Following embolization, the fibroids typically become soft and squishy. This change is like the difference between having a firm rubber ball sitting on your bladder and then having a Nerf ball of the same size sitting on your bladder. Studies describing early results of UAE suggested that the amount of volume reduction following UAE does not correlate with the amount of symptom relief.[10] In other words, women experience greater relief in their symptoms than would be expected from how much the volume of the uterus decreased, suggesting that this composition change is important.

Even so, studies examining long-term outcomes suggest that volume reduction is critical for achieving symptom relief. In a series of women treated in the United States and followed for 5 years, more than 70 percent were happy with their results at 5 years.[11] Women with symptom control at 1 year were more than five times as likely to have symptom control at 5 years.

In this study, UAE failed to control symptoms more than twice as often in women with a larger uterus.[11] Taking all the uterine volumes and ranking them by size and looking at the larger group versus the smaller group, the midpoint (median) was 717 cm³, or the size the uterus would be with about a 10- to 11-cm fibroid or several fibroids equivalent to this volume (as in table 11.1, which shows that a 10-cm fibroid has a volume of 525 cm³, and a 15-cm fibroid has a volume of 1,814 cm³, so 717 cm³ appears consistent with a little bigger than 10).

A study from France found that not only increased volume but also an increased number of fibroids led to less success.[12] A rule of thumb emerged from this study which says that for each 1 cm in a leiomyoma's diameter at baseline, the chance of failure increased by a factor of about one and a half.[12] Similarly, for each additional fibroid present prior to treatment, the chance of failure increased by about one and a third.[12]

Several other factors influence the success of UAE. First, if only one uterine artery can be embolized, the procedure often will not work. The uterus easily establishes its blood supply from the remaining artery. Second, if the fibroid receives its major blood supply from another blood vessel, such as the ovarian or cervical artery, then embolizing the uterine arteries does not produce good results.[13] The appearance of the fibroids on magnetic resonance imaging (MRI) generally predicts success[10,14]; fibroids that appear dark on T2 weighted images appear to respond best. Finally, degenerated fibroids (fibroids that have previously lost their blood supply) do not respond to UAE; these fibroids have had a "natural UAE."

Together these results suggest that, like laparoscopic and hysteroscopic myomectomy, UAE is best performed in women who have a limited number of fibroids and fibroids that are smaller. We clearly need interventions with fewer side effects to treat women earlier than we do now. Many diseases in the past were treated surgically at a very advanced state and can now be treated earlier. Breast cancer has been transformed from a disease in which a large mass in the breast was the first sign, to a disease frequently treated when there is an abnormal mammogram and the cancer is too small to feel.

Likewise, hernias used to be treated when there was a big bulge in the abdominal wall, and now they are repaired at the first sign of abdominal wall weakness. We have a long way to go with fibroids.

Pregnancy and Childbearing after UAE

Uterine artery embolization generally is recommended for women who do not wish to have future pregnancies.[15] A number of women have had successful pregnancies following UAE, however, and many of them were in their forties when they had the UAE, meaning they already had an increased risk of infertility and pregnancy complications based on their age.[16–19]

One reason for this recommendation is that the UAE procedure affects the blood supply to the ovaries. If the main blood supply to the uterus is cut off via the uterine arteries, then the uterus tries to get a blood supply from the smaller blood vessels that supply it, called the *collateral blood vessels*, to keep itself alive. The most important collateral blood supply to the uterus is the ovarian arteries. Although some people argue that ovarian function should be affected only if the embolic particles are incorrectly targeted and hit the ovaries, understanding the blood supply to the uterus tells us that even with correct targeting, blood flow to the ovaries can be interrupted. The uterus is a smart organ; if one area of blood supply is cut off, another will be recruited to replace it.

This effect on ovarian function is seen most clearly in women who stop having periods following UAE (again, technically this is called amenorrhea). Early studies described rates of amenorrhea of 5 to 8 percent following UAE and reported that, like women undergoing chemotherapy, sometimes women would resume having regular periods later.[5,20] The largest study (consisting of more than 500 women) suggests that the risk of amenorrhea is age-related.[19,21] For women under age 40 the risk of amenorrhea is only 3 percent, whereas for women over 50 the risk is 40 percent. In several cases the woman's level of the hormone FSH rose, like it does in menopause when the periods stop, suggesting that the procedure caused a transient menopause-like state.[22,23]

This finding makes sense, since older women have less "ovarian reserve" as they approach the age of natural menopause. Since the average age of menopause is 51 in the United States, women still menstruating after that age likely are close to menopause anyway. For women who desire fertility, however, the number of women who have such severe ovarian damage that they stop having periods is only the tip of the iceberg. A major cause of infertility in women as they age is decreased ovarian reserve, having fewer eggs, or a less good quality egg, which makes getting pregnant harder. Thus, the number of women with ovarian damage may be significantly underestimated by concentrating only on those who stop having periods. I think of the risk of ovarian damage like a triangle (or iceberg): the top is women who stop having periods, but the base is women with normal cycles who have trouble getting pregnant.

Although there have been reports of women who got pregnant following UAE-induced amenorrhea, no one has followed a large group of women attempting pregnancy after UAE.[18] Therefore we do not know whether failing to become pregnant or having difficulty getting pregnant is a major issue or not. However, if 3 percent of young women have enough of a shock to the ovary to stop having periods, even temporarily, how many may have fertility problems later due to lost eggs? Longer-term studies are necessary. There has been a report of one woman who stopped having periods after UAE but who nevertheless had normal ovarian function.[24] In this case the endometrium (uterine lining) appeared to be affected by the UAE.

Each individual and her doctor need to make a decision together regarding UAE and plans for pregnancy. For women with an increased risk of surgical complications, like someone with a previous myomectomy, the risks of UAE may be very acceptable. Or, for some women, the benefit of a quicker recovery may be more important than a possible decrease in fertility. Finally, deciding whether optimizing the chance of pregnancy is the critical point or instead just making sure the door to pregnancy is left open is an important distinction when deciding on newer therapies such as UAE, in which the longer-term results are unknown. Only with more and longer studies will we have real answers.

In addition to a number of reports of normal pregnancy, cases have been reported of significant pregnancy complications following UAE.[16,17,25] Again, because large series of women have not been followed from UAE through pregnancy, we do not know whether this is a rare event or a common one. We need to know both the numerator (the number of women having pregnancy complications) and the denominator (the total number of women undergoing UAE and attempting pregnancy) of this important fraction.

There is also a bias toward reporting pregnancy complications; medical journals are not interested in normal pregnancies following a procedure. If a woman has an unusual complication, her doctor has greater motivation to write about this rare event. Nonetheless, because some of the embolic particles likely end up damaging the normal uterus, there is reason to believe that pregnancy complications could be increased after UAE.

In one large study in Canada in which women were followed as a cohort following UAE (so we get both numerator and denominator), again healthy pregnancies did occur, but there were also a greater than expected number of problems with the placenta.[19] Twelve percent of women had abnormal placentation, either placenta previa (whereby the placenta implants over the cervical opening, blocking vaginal delivery and putting the woman at risk for severe bleeding) or placenta accreta (whereby the placenta embeds itself too deeply in the uterine wall and does not separate easily following delivery). This is a high percentage of women having this problem, and none of these women had had previous pregnancies (abnormal placentation more often occurs in women who have had prior deliveries or cesarean sections or both). These placenta problems also fit what we know about the risks, in theory, of the procedure; if the normal uterine wall is partially embolized, then damage may occur to the wall like it does during C-section. Clearly women contemplating pregnancy following UAE and their obstetricians need to be aware of this risk.

It has been argued that UAE has long been done for women shortly after delivery for problems such as postpartum hemorrhage and that the results are good. Although the procedure is similar, the situations are entirely different. Bleeding immediately after pregnancy is usually caused by an abnormality of the placenta, an inability of the uterus to contract normally, or a change in blood-clotting factors due to excessive bleeding. These events are transient, and the situation would not be the same a week or a month later. Having a 6- to 10-cm mass in the uterine wall (a fibroid) is a stable cause of bleeding, however, and thus comparing the two situations may not be valid. The blood supply to the uterus is also enhanced during pregnancy. All the collateral blood supply we discussed earlier is recruited during pregnancy and is ready and better able to support the uterus following blockage of the uterine arteries when UAE is performed during or following pregnancy.

Potential Complications

Life-threatening complications have been reported following UAE, but they are rare.[26] In an initial series of studies comparing patients undergoing surgery and patients undergoing UAE, the risk of major complications following UAE appeared to be lower than with traditional surgeries.[8,27] There are now four randomized clinical trials comparing UAE with hysterectomy (two studies), myomectomy (one study), or both (one study), which together suggest that the rate of major complications is the same.[28–32]

A Cochrane Review (the authoritative source for evidence-based medicine) of these studies concludes that UAE is associated with a shorter hospital stay and a faster return to work. It is also associated with more minor complications, unscheduled visits, and higher readmission rates. UAE and surgery have similar rates of complications, but the type and timing of complications differ.

The study that randomized women to UAE or surgery (with 15 percent of women having myomectomy and 85 percent hysterectomy) has reported outcomes one year following treatment.[32] Although both groups had equivalent quality of life at one year, 9 percent of women in the embolization group required another procedure (a second embolization or a hysterectomy).

These studies will continue to give us important information as women are followed longer and additional information is reported in the scientific literature. It will be important to learn whether UAE treatment failures mainly occur during the first year or whether 9 percent of women have additional procedures every year. It will also be critical to know whether symptomatic relief is equivalent with myomectomy and UAE. (Although the symptom scores were lower in the surgery group in the reported trial, this may not be a fair comparison; it is hard to have fibroid symptoms when you no longer have a uterus.)[32]

It is important to note that all these trials took place outside the United States, so all the information may not be applicable to women in this country. With universal health care systems in Europe, women may have less freedom to choose their therapy. Most important, black women may not be well represented in these trials. The racial make-up of the participants in the study reporting one-year outcomes was not described, but given the study sites, it is likely that they were mainly Caucasian.[32]

It will be important as new treatments are introduced that funding is available for trials here and that women participate in trials that allow them to be randomly assigned to a treatment option. Although it is hard to decide to enter a trial and to lose control of deciding on your own treatment, if incomplete information is available on which to make your decision, this is a reasonable option that will also benefit others in the future.

In addition to postembolization syndrome (discussed above), another well-known minor complication is that women with submucosal fibroids frequently expel the necrotic (dead) fibroids through the cervix and vagina.[8,33,34] It is not possible to predict the timing of when women will experience this complication. It can occur several days following the UAE or even a year later.[8] This outcome can be beneficial because it increases the volume reduction following UAE, but women often experience laborlike pain when the fibroid dilates the cervix, and the risk of infection is increased. Thus, most experts consider hysteroscopic myomectomy to be a better technique for treatment of a Type 0 or I fibroid, and UAE and hysteroscopic myomectomy complementary, and not competing, techniques.

Encouraged by the success of UAE for the treatment of fibroids, gynecologists are performing several new procedures that try to surgically mimic the effect of UAE. These include surgeries such as laparoscopy, which tie off the uterine arteries,[35] and approaches that use a clamp on the cervix to compress the arteries for several hours.[36] The drawback of these approaches is that there are other vital structures near the uterine arteries, particularly the ureters, that can be damaged. Although UAE causes a small risk of damage to the blood vessels, it does not carry risk of injury to adjacent structures in the way that these other techniques may. Also, since some of these techniques require surgery, the standard surgical risks are added to the risk of vascular occlusion. Clearly, these approaches require further study.

I believe UAE will continue to be a treatment used for the near future. Although its use for women who desire future fertility is controversial, for a woman with no plans for pregnancy, it gives relief of both bleeding and bulk symptoms in a minimally invasive fashion. There is also a small subgroup of women who view the ovarian impairment as an advantage. For women in their fifties who have been trying to temporize until menopause for years, having UAE bring on menopause can be desirable rather than a drawback.

CHAPTER 12

Focused Ultrasound Surgery and Other Thermoablative Therapies

Many efforts have been made to try to find less invasive ways to destroy fibroids. Most of the less invasive techniques that have been developed involve either thermoablative therapies or image-guided therapy or both.

Thermoablative therapies use heat or cold to destroy tissue. This approach has been used in the treatment of other diseases, including freezing the cervix to treat abnormal Pap smears and using a variety of probes to heat lesions in organs such as the liver or the kidneys.

Image-guided therapy involves the use of some type of imaging to guide the procedure, rather than a traditional surgical (visualize and touch) approach.[1] The imaging can be provided by conventional X-rays, ultrasound, or more sophisticated methods, such as computed tomography (CT) or magnetic resonance imaging (MRI) guidance. Some of these techniques have been around for many years, such as the use of dye and X-rays to examine the uterus and the fallopian tubes when a hysterosalpingogram is done as a part of a fertility workup. Many are relatively new, such as CT guidance used to drain abscesses deep in the body without open surgery.

One of the earliest approaches for uterine fibroids using a thermoablative technique utilized a probe to deliver heat during a conventional surgical approach. Myolysis (as discussed in Chapter 9) was first introduced using a laser; in further studies bipolar needles were used to destroy the fibroid tissue.[2,3] Both of these devices were used at the time of laparoscopy to destroy a subserosal or intramural fibroid without literally excising it, as would be done at the time of a laparoscopic myomectomy. The advantage of this approach is that less finely tuned surgical skills were needed than for one that utilized laparoscopic suturing. This circumstance would make a laparoscopic approach available for more women undergoing surgery, but it still required a surgical approach and general anesthesia.

Myolysis was never widely accepted, likely for several reasons. First of all, from a physician's point of view, the procedure was rather tedious, and even a small fibroid needed multiple placements of the probe to destroy it. Concerns were also raised about the risk of adhesions or scar tissue that would form on the surface after this approach. There were also procedures done using a freezing probe (cryomyolysis) in a similar manner at the time of surgery.[4] This technique did not gain wide acceptance, probably for similar reasons.

The next wave in these minimally invasive therapies came when MRI monitoring could be used for control of therapy. This was an important development, since there are special MRI parameters that can gauge temperature. The problem with surgical control of thermoablative therapies is that the eye has to gauge when the correct temperature is reached and the procedure is complete. This is as difficult to do as gauging the temperature of a pot sitting on the stove by looking at it. Clearly, you can get some clues by direct vision, such as when steam is emitted from the pot, but an accurate visual gauge is impossible.

Accurate gauging of the temperature created during a thermoablative therapy is critical. If the temperature is too high, normal tissue is likely to be damaged or destroyed. This can present safety problems and can lead to injury of other tissue, in addition to the previously discussed risk of adhesions. However, if the peak temperature is too low, the tissue may not be destroyed, and, in essence, there is no effective treatment. This is a particular issue for fibroid treatments because fibroids vary widely in their composition and the same amount of energy does not produce the same target temperature or amount of tissue destruction in every fibroid.

The first image-guided thermoablative therapy for fibroids was conducted in a small series of patients who underwent cryomyolysis during laparoscopy performed in a special MRI machine that allowed surgical procedures to be carried out while the patient was in the MRI magnet.[5,6] However this MRI-guided cryomyolysis required both the traditional surgical incisions and treatment within an MRI machine and also has not been widely adopted. Not only was this approach more costly and just as invasive, but many traditional surgical instruments are metal and can't be used in an MRI machine.

A later approach, percutaneous laser ablation, involved inserting laser fibers through the skin of the abdominal wall and into the targeted fibroid. Only local anesthesia was used during this procedure; it was used to numb the skin where the fibers were inserted.[7,8] After the fibers were in the fibroid, treatment took place while the woman was inside a standard MRI machine so that the temperature could be gauged. Although this laser ablation approach was limited to fibroids in the front of the uterus, the approach was much less invasive and allowed women to be treated as outpatients; follow-up at one year demonstrated shrinkage of the treated fibroid and a decrease in menstrual blood loss following treatment.[8]

Using focused ultrasound instead of the laser fibers led to the first noninvasive thermoablative therapy, MRI-guided focused ultrasound surgery (MRgFUS).[9-12] This is the only thermoablative therapy for uterine fibroids that has received the approval of the Food and Drug Administration (FDA).

Focused ultrasound surgery (FUS) and *high intensity focused ultrasound* (HIFU) are two terms that describe a similar process. Just like a magnifying glass can focus light so that heat can be produced at a specific point, multiple ultrasound waves can pass through the skin at different points and only at the focal point where they all meet will they deliver enough energy to cause tissue destruction (fig. 12.1). By using many different bursts of these focused ultrasound waves, a fibroid can be destroyed. Each individual burst of FUS energy is termed a *sonication* (sonic = sound).

The MRI guidance allows the temperature of the treated fibroid to be measured during each sonication to maximize complete treatment and minimize injury to surrounding structures. In addition, the MRI provides a view of all the important structures around the uterus (like the bowel, bladder, and pelvic nerves) and thus helps to avoid injury to these structures.

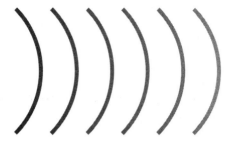

Typical diagnostic ultrasound waves

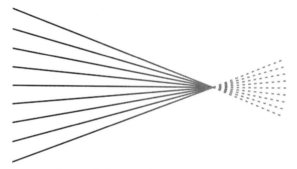

Focused ultrasound waves

Figure 12.1. Both diagnostic ultrasound and focused ultrasound surgery (FUS) use similar frequencies of ultrasound energy. Just as light can be used to see structures, or multiple waves of light can be harnessed in a laser to destroy tissue, ultrasound can be used in various ways. In diagnostic ultrasound, the waves of ultrasound move out from a transducer, hit their target (the fibroid or the baby's face in the case of prenatal ultrasound), and produce a picture of the target. With focused ultrasound, each individual ultrasound wave has so little energy that it can pass through intervening structures (like the skin) without damage. Only where multiple waves converge is there enough energy to cause damage. At the focus in FUS, the temperature will briefly reach 60 to 80 degrees Centigrade, in contrast to the normal body temperature of 37 degrees Centigrade. Some energy continues past the focus (illustrated by dotted lines), so the areas both in front of and behind the focus need to be examined to perform this procedure safely.

During treatment a woman is lying on her stomach so that her fibroid is up against the source of the ultrasound energy, which is in the bed of the MRI. Generally an intravenous line is inserted so the woman can have some pain medication and relaxing drugs similar to those used in UAE. A catheter is used to empty her bladder so the fibroid does not move as the bladder fills during the treatment; the catheter also eliminates the need for the woman to use the bathroom, which would require stopping the treatment. The woman is also asked to shave the top part of her pubic hair prior to the procedure, since this decreases skin burns caused by tiny air bubbles trapped at the base of the hairs. Most programs also use elastic stockings to keep the blood from pooling in the legs while the woman is lying still for treatment, preventing deep vein thromboses (DVTs) and pulmonary embolisms (PEs), similar to the procedures used during surgical approaches.

Treatment currently takes place over about 3 hours. Because there are no incisions and the sedation is light, women go home after treatment. Most women go back to work in 1 or 2 days, with 4 days the longest reported time out of work in the studies.[12]

In contrast to UAE, women having FUS treatment typically do not have the pain and fever of postembolization syndrome after treatment. There appears to be a difference between the ischemic necrosis caused when the blood supply to the uterus is interrupted following UAE and the coagulative necrosis caused by FUS, in which the proteins are immediately denatured (like the changes that occur when cooking an egg). With ischemic necrosis, cells are broken open as they die and release agents that cause fever; this process does not occur with coagulative necrosis. Although initially it was not clear whether there was a difference between the two types of necrosis or just the amount of tissue treated, it is now clear there is a difference in the type of necrosis.

There appear to be parallels between UAE and FUS, however, in that both provide at least some of their short-term symptom relief without necessarily causing shrinkage. To provide a variation on the analogy used in Chapter 11, having a lead ball sitting on your bladder is more uncomfortable than having a cotton ball of the same size in the same place.

Early studies have shown that between 70 and 80 percent of women have at least a 10-point improvement in symptoms at 6 months as determined by the Symptom Severity Score (SSS) of the Uterine Fibroid Symptoms Quality of Life (UFS-QOL) questionnaire.[11–13] This measure is important for the studies of FUS and is likely to be used in assessment of more fibroid treatments in the future.

Quality of life is more difficult to measure than the amount of shrinkage of a fibroid achieved by ultrasound treatment, but it is more important. How a disease affects your life and work is what matters. Many standard questionnaires look at health-related quality of life. A good summary of the field is found at www.cdc.gov/hrqol.

The UFS-QOL is the only questionnaire that specifically asks questions about both the bleeding symptoms and the bulk-related symptoms experienced by women with uterine fibroids.[13] There are several different parts of the UFS-QOL; the most widely used is the Symptom Severity Score. The SSS uses 8 questions to understand how much the symptoms of fibroids affect a woman's quality of life. It is scored on a 100-point scale; normal women usually score around 20 points, and women with fibroids score on average 40 points.[13] Thus, when the studies were designed to test focused ultrasound treatment (termed the *pivotal trial*), a 10-point improvement appeared to be a meaningful measure of fibroid symptom improvement. Women in the focused ultrasound studies who improved only 8 points would be considered treatment failures. This is a higher bar than that used in most other fibroid studies including those of UAE, in which even 1 point of improvement could count as improvement or the target could be a 10 percent improvement (4 points if the baseline is 40 points). "Success rates" between different studies cannot be compared if they are not measuring the same thing.

In fact, a 10-point improvement proved to be a conservative estimate of improvement in the initial study of FUS. Women enrolled in this trial had a baseline SSS of over 60 before treatment and on average had more than 20 points of improvement 6 months following treatment.[12] Modest shrinkage of the treated fibroid was also seen at 6 months, on average 13 percent, with treatment of an average of 10 percent of the total amount of fibroid(s) in the uterus.[12]

One of the issues that need to be assessed in early reports of new technologies is whether the drug or device is FDA-approved for use in treating another disease or condition (an indication for treatment). If there is no approved indication, all treatments will take place as a part of clinical trials regulated by the FDA because the drug or device is "investigational." However, in the United States (but not in most other countries), individual physicians are allowed to use approved agents for treatments of other indications if there is sound medical evidence that they may be safe and effective.

Focused ultrasound had no other approved indication, and thus all women were enrolled in the clinical trials. Only by participating in the FDA-supervised trials could women and doctors have access to treatment. In contrast, when UAE was evolving, the catheters and the embolic agents it utilized were available to treat other diseases, and doctors were allowed to use them "off label" for fibroids. Treatment is more likely to be conservative in trials of technology with no approved indication.

The FUS clinical trials were thus designed to maximize safety, since this technique was new. In the first group of patients treated for the FDA approval, a maximum of 150 cm^3 of tissue (about 6.5 × 6.5 × 6.5 cm) was able to be treated under FDA study rules. This is why on average only 10 percent of the total volume of fibroids present in the uterus was able to be treated.[12] Aiming for 80 percent treatment in the first trial would not optimize safety.

It is reasonable to expect that better long-term results will be achieved with more complete fibroid treatment, as has been demonstrated with UAE. When we look at patients treated under more liberal treatment guidelines as the process from initial FDA review to commercial approval for FUS moved forward, it appears that women receiving more extensive treatments have lower symptom severity scores.[14]

Because FUS did not receive approval from the FDA until 2005, however, we do not yet have much long-term data on symptom relief at this time. However, all women are being followed for 3 years, and additional information will be published. We will probably find that some individuals benefit more than others from FUS and also that additional treatment may be needed for new fibroids. Nevertheless, the noninvasive nature of the treatment will likely make it a good option for women in the future.

Who is currently a candidate for FUS treatment? The FDA labeling of the device reports that FUS is intended for premenopausal women with symptomatic fibroids who have no plans for future pregnancy. In general, a volume of about a 10 × 10 × 10 cm fibroid can be treated in a single session.

Currently a detailed MRI with gadolinium is performed prior to treatment to assess a number of important factors, including the location of the fibroid in relation to the bowel, bladder, and major pelvic nerves. Treatment is not undertaken if a significant amount of energy would hit any of these vital structures and cause damage. The software program of the device allows the surgeon to calculate the energy delivered at each point to avoid this complication.

Gadolinium is a substance that lights up any area of the body with blood flow during an MRI. Thus, a small amount is placed in the bloodstream through an IV site before MRIs to see whether the blood supply is cut off in parts of the uterus. Both FUS and UAE appear to be significantly less effective if there is not good blood supply to the fibroid prior to treatment. Fibroids without blood supply have in effect gone through a "natural UAE." Gadolinium is also used after FUS treatment to assess how effective the treatment was in devascularizing (cutting off the blood supply) of the tissue.

Recording the position of any abdominal wall scars and avoiding them during treatment is an important part of treatment planning. Scars have a lot of extracellular matrix (ECM), just as fibroids do, and this makes them absorb more energy than normal skin. This energy absorption by scars is painful for women and also makes the treatment less effective, since not all the energy reaches the target. Most important, it appears that sending focused ultrasound energy through the scar may make the patient susceptible to significant skin burns, as has been reported in one case.[15]

Data from all treatments are recorded; this allows subsequent retrospective analysis, which has helped to decrease complications for future treatments. A nerve injury reported in the pivotal trial resulted in reversible pain and weakness in the woman's leg following treatment. The analysis determined that the nerve was not directly injured but that part of the pelvic bone was heated.[12] Bone absorbs heat more readily than soft tissue (just as a roast with a bone inside will cook faster than the same piece of meat without a bone), and thus the bone passively delivered heat to the nerve. Since that time the distance to the bone has become part of treatment planning.

In addition, the treatment software allows the surgeon to change and regulate the treatment at any point. Before going to a high-energy sonication for treatment, he or she can use a low-energy "test sonication" to make sure that the targeting is correct and the patient is comfortable. Also, some fibroids are homogeneous and require the same energy level throughout the treatment. In other fibroids there is significant variation, and therefore the power needs to be adjusted many times during the procedure to maximize both safety and efficacy. The patient and doctor communicate throughout the procedure to help assess her comfort and safety.

The indications for treatment for FUS may change substantially over time as experience is gained with the technique. Already studies have been reported using gonadotropin-releasing hormone (GnRH) agonists to shrink fibroids before treatment, and studies are under way regarding whether FUS is an appropriate treatment for women who plan future pregnancies.[16]

The fact that FUS is a fibroid-specific therapy may be an advantage for women seeking fertility. It has the potential to destroy the fibroid directly without injuring the normal myometrium. FUS is also being investigated for use in the treatment of many other diseases, including cancerous tumors. My hope is that the noninvasive nature of this technology might allow early intervention for fibroids and potentially even prevention in the future.

Technology is also likely to change this therapy and even introduce new therapies over the next few years. Just as computers process data faster (and become less expensive) over time, technological advances can change FUS significantly so that more fibroids can be treated in the same amount of time or the same amount of fibroids can be treated faster. Similarly, we have seen laparoscopy evolve from being used simply to perform tubal ligations to being used to perform supracervical hysterectomies. FUS, too, is a rapidly changing field.

Some studies have worked with an ultrasound-guided FUS system.[17–20] In this device, conventional ultrasound monitors the procedure via a transabdominal approach and a vaginal probe that delivers the FUS energy to the uterus. This system is designed to treat submucosal fibroids. The limitation of the system to date has been the lack of thermal monitoring and the potential for vaginal burns.[20] This system has not yet been tested in clinical trials for women.

CHAPTER 13

Hysterectomy

Why would any woman choose to have a hysterectomy today when so many alternatives are available? For a woman with fibroids, there are several reasons. The first is that hysterectomy provides a cure for uterine fibroids and eliminates the problem of recurrent fibroids. If a woman wants to eliminate her risk of fibroid symptoms in the future, hysterectomy is currently her only choice.

Second, hysterectomy also cures a number of other problems that can coexist with fibroids. Conditions such as adenomyosis, endometriosis, and endometrial polyps can cause some of the symptoms being attributed to the fibroids. Other conditions that are not related to fibroids—such as cervical dysplasia (a precancerous condition detected by abnormal Pap smears)—may be best treated with hysterectomy, which simultaneously eliminates the fibroids and these unrelated problems.

Finally, studies show that hysterectomy improves the quality of life for most women with fibroids.[1–6]

There are sometimes good reasons for a woman to have a hysterectomy. However, hysterectomy is a major surgical procedure. It requires either a general anesthesia or a spinal or epidural anesthesia. It requires staying in the hospital at least a day and possibly several days. Depending on the size of the uterus, hysterectomy requires at least a vaginal incision and, usually for women with fibroids, one or more abdominal incisions, as well. There are also risks of postoperative anemia (sometimes requiring transfusion), infection, and other typical complications of surgery, although serious complications are rare.[7,8] (Most reports of complications following hysterectomy include women undergoing this procedure for cancer as well women with fibroids. Women with cancer have higher rates of complications.)

Some data suggest that vaginal hysterectomies result in fewer complications than abdominal ones.[9] However, a woman who has a very large uterus or who has had multiple prior surgeries, and who therefore would not be eligible for a vaginal hysterectomy, may be at risk for additional complications. The decreased risk of complications for a vaginal hysterectomy may be less related to the surgical approach per se and more related to the physiological characteristics of the woman who is eligible to undergo this procedure. Only a study in which women with similar uteruses are randomly assigned to the two types of hysterectomy would help us understand the different outcomes. Complications for abdominal hysterectomies appear to be increased in women with larger uteruses.[10]

A *total abdominal hysterectomy* (TAH) removes both the fundus (top) of the uterus and the cervix (fig. 13.1). Leaving the cervix in place is termed a *supracervical* (above the cervix) hysterectomy (SCH) or *subtotal hysterectomy*. In a vaginal *hysterectomy* (VH), the cervix is generally removed because it *is* difficult to remove the uterus from a vaginal approach without first removing the cervix. Removing the ovaries is normally considered a second procedure, a *bilateral salpingo-oophorectomy* (BSO), meaning removal of both (bilateral) ovaries (oophorectomy) and fallopian tubes (salpingectomy).

Types of Hysterectomy

Several types of hysterectomy are available. The terminology can be somewhat confusing, and it is easiest to think about the options in the following way:

1. Will the ovaries be removed or left in place?
2. Will the cervix be removed with the rest of the uterus or left in place?
3. What type of incision(s) will need to be made to remove this uterus?

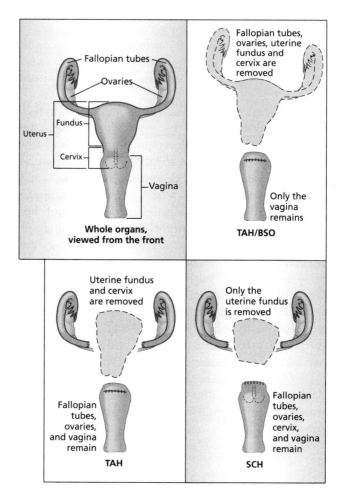

Figure 13.1. Different types of hysterectomies, with the structures removed shown with dashed lines and the pelvis at the end of the surgery drawn normally. In a total abdominal hysterectomy with bilateral salpingo-oophorectomy (TAH/BSO), the entire uterus (both fundus and cervix), fallopian tubes, and ovaries are all removed. Because the vagina must be entered to remove the cervix, the top of the vagina has been sutured. Although the pelvis appears "empty" in this drawing, both the large and small intestines fill this space. In a total abdominal hysterectomy (TAH), the fundus and the cervix (in other words, the "total" uterus) are removed, but the ovaries and tubes are left behind. The attachments of the ovaries and tubes to the uterus are removed, but their major support and blood supply still remain from the side of the bony pelvis. In a supracervical, or subtotal, hysterectomy (SCH), the cervix, ovaries, and tubes are left behind. Generally the top of the cervix is closed at the time of surgery, so there is no passageway between the vagina and the pelvic cavity.

Will the ovaries be removed or left in place?

The ovaries generally are not removed when a hysterectomy is performed for uterine fibroids. Removing the uterus alone will cure the bleeding and the size-related symptoms caused by the fibroids. Removing the ovaries is thus not required in treating fibroids as it is for other diseases like endometriosis or gynecologic cancers.

Many physicians were taught that at a set age (which varies between 35 and 50) women should be told that removal of the ovaries is recommended as part of the surgery, in the mode of "while we are there, we may as well." The general teaching had been that ovaries don't have any function after menopause and the risk of ovarian cancer increases with increasing age, so removing the ovaries near the time of menopause was a no-lose proposition. This was especially true if hormone replacement therapy could be used to help younger women transition to the time when they would naturally go through menopause.

However, more recent research suggests that although after menopause the ovaries don't make much estradiol (the major estrogen in premenopausal women), they make a tremendous amount of androgens (usually thought of as male hormones).[11] It is thought that these androgens may be important in maintaining mood and sex drive.[12-14] In addition, the risks of hormone replacement have become clearer, and many fewer women choose to use hormones following menopause.[15,16] (Most women are aware that there has been research from the Women's Health Initiative demonstrating significant complications with postmenopausal hormone replacement therapy. However, it is not widely known that the risks are lower for women without a uterus, who are able to take estrogen alone.)[16] Recently the role of prematurely losing the ovaries in increasing the risk of heart disease has also been explored.[17]

Considering all these factors, there are good reasons to retain the ovaries if possible. The major reason to remove them at the time of fibroid surgery is if the woman has a high risk of ovarian cancer. There are several Internet-based sites that help women assess their risk of ovarian cancer—the Women's Cancer Network (www.wcn.org), for example. There is also strong evidence that removing the uterus, even if the ovaries are left in place, reduces the risk of ovarian cancer.[18,19] (A similar reduction in ovarian cancer risk is seen in women who have had a tubal ligation, suggesting that there is some kind of molecular communication between the uterus and ovaries.) Thus, unless they have a high risk of ovarian cancer, many women choose to keep their ovaries when undergoing a hysterectomy for fibroids.

Should the cervix be removed with the rest of the uterus?

Just as with the ovaries, the cervix does not need to be removed to remedy the symptoms caused by uterine fibroids. In fact, in the era before we had good antibiotics, the cervix was routinely not removed because removing it would entail entering the vagina, which leads to an increased risk of postoperative infection. (The vagina, just like the mouth, is filled with bacteria.) However, with better antibiotics, the trend became to remove the cervix to prevent cancer of the cervix from developing. Supracervical hysterectomy has only recently come back into practice.[20]

The development of the Pap smear (named for its inventor, Dr. George Papanicolau) has made it less necessary to remove the cervix during hysterectomy. The Pap smear became one of the most important early detection and prevention tools for any cancer ever seen. A Pap smear involves using a small brush or spatula (or both) to gently collect cells on the surface of the cervix so they can be viewed under a microscope. Not only can cancerous cells be detected early, when treatment options are better, but precancerous cells can be detected and treated, so that cancer is prevented. These precancerous cells, called *cervical dysplasia*, can be frozen, burned, or surgically removed. Increasingly, tests for human papilloma virus (HPV), which is thought to cause cervical cancer, can also be used to predict who is most at risk for developing cervical cancer. (A vaccine to prevent HPV infection is being introduced and is likely to have a big impact on this disease in the future.)

The major reason for removing the cervix at the time of hysterectomy for fibroids continues to be eliminating the possibility of cancer of the cervix. This risk is very low, however, if the woman has never had an abnormal Pap smear and is in a mutually monogamous relationship (neither she nor her sex partner has additional partners, which eliminates new exposure to HPV). This risk is also low if women continue to get Pap smears or HPV testing (or both) as recommended following SCH. However, many women do not receive this routine preventive care and may be less motivated to get Pap smears once their fibroid problems are resolved with hysterectomy.

It is also possible that new fibroids could develop in the cervix if it is left behind. This has never been reported but could occur.

An argument for retaining the cervix is that it may be important for sexual function and pelvic support. Clearly the cervix is stimulated during vaginal intercourse, and removing it changes the vagina and leaves some scar tissue where the cervix was removed. Early studies suggested that women had improved sexual function following SCH, but generally no comparison group was studied. However, a recent randomized clinical trial in which half the women were randomly assigned to SCH and the other half to TAH suggests that sexual function is the same, at least up to two years following surgery.[21] Other studies suggest that preoperative sexual function and depression are important determinants of sexual function after hysterectomy. For most women without depression, sexual function improves following definitive resolution of symptoms.[22,23]

Problems with pelvic support following hysterectomy cause the bladder, bowel, and vagina to bulge downward, or prolapse. To understand prolapse, it helps to visualize the uterus like an upside-down pear suspended in the middle of a large mixing bowl (fig. 13.2). The bowl represents the pelvic bones, and the pear represents the uterus with cervix. There are two pairs of tough fibrous bands that keep the uterus in place by connecting the bony pelvis and the cervix. The cardinal ligaments go out from either side of the cervix and attach to the sides of the pelvis. The uterosacral ligaments go out from the cervix, go around the bowel, and hold the cervix to the sacrum, the part of the pelvis analogous to the back of the bowl. These attachments provide the major structural support of the uterus.

If the cervix is left in place, the cardinal and uterosacral ligaments remain. If the cervix is removed, these ligaments are cut and sutured where they attach to the cervix. Women worry that after a hysterectomy they will have a big "hole" in the pelvis where the uterus and cervix used to be. There is no hole after surgery because the bowel and bladder, which are also located in the pelvis, naturally expand to fill the space where the uterus and cervix had been. The bowel and bladder regularly expand and contract in size with normal bowel and bladder function. These organs have more freedom to occupy the middle of the pelvis following hysterectomy.

If the cervix is removed and these ligaments are cut, the bowel, bladder, and rectum, which rest on the cervix or lower part of the

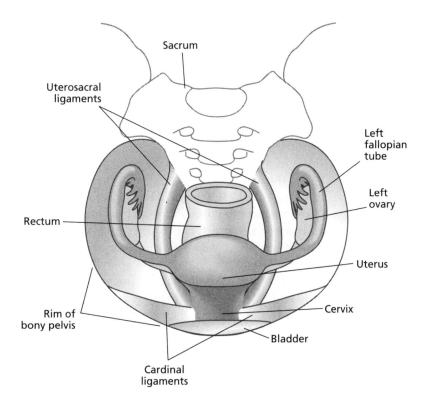

Figure 13.2. The uterus is similar in shape to an upside-down pear. It is pictured here in the bowl-like pelvis. The uterus does not float freely but is anchored at several points. The cardinal ligaments go straight out from the cervix to attach to the side of the pelvis. The uterosacral ligaments start at the point where the cervix joins the fundus. They swing out and back to attach to the bony pelvis behind the uterus. This is where the spine is located and is called the sacrum.

uterus, may be pulled downward by the force of gravity over time. This has historically been a major problem following hysterectomy. However, these ligaments also tend to be stretched during childbirth, and in the past women had more children and more vaginal deliveries than women do today. Thus, it is not clear whether this risk will be the same for women in the future as it has been in the past. There is also increasing evidence that particular women with less strong collagen or problems with extracellular matrix (ECM) may have an increased risk of prolapse.

The randomized clinical trial comparing TAH and SCH can guide us on this issue, as well. This study reported that women who underwent SCH had fewer intraoperative complications and a quicker recovery than women undergoing a TAH.[24] However, approximately 7 percent of women who had an SCH had some sort of cyclic bleeding.[24] This cyclic bleeding is typically spotting or staining and is much less heavy than a normal period, but it occurs at the same time (monthly) in response to the changes in the ovarian hormones that cause normal periods. Over the first year there were no differences in bladder functioning or prolapse, but there were a few women in the SCH group who had prolapse of their cervix.[24] Finally, over the first two years of follow-up there was improved quality of life and sexual functioning (as we discussed previously) in both groups.[21]

Most doctors believe that the reason for cyclic bleeding following SCH is that some of the endometrial lining in the uterus was left behind with the cervix. For that reason, many gynecologists will remove the innermost part of the cervix at the same time. However, there is some recent evidence that the cervix may respond to hormones, as well, and this may be a complication that cannot be avoided. Thus, the randomized study was important in uncovering new issues not seen in prior studies of hysterectomy.

There is no one-size-fits-all answer to the question of whether the cervix should be removed for the woman who is at low risk for cervical cancer. The studies looking at short-term sexual function and prolapse suggest that SCH is not as beneficial as previously supposed. However, for a woman who undergoes a hysterectomy in her thirties or forties, the real concern is not two years down the road but decades later.

Until we have long-term outcome studies, every woman will need to make her own choice based on individual factors. A woman who unfailingly goes for routine preventive medical care is a better candidate for an SCH than a woman who is unlikely to go for a Pap smear every few years following SCH. Likewise, if pressure against the cervix is a critical part of a woman's sexual response, an SCH may be a better choice.

I counsel women that there is a chance of forming cervical fibroids following a supracervical hysterectomy, although this is likely a very small risk. Rarely, the cervix later needs to be surgically removed in a separate procedure (termed a *trachelectomy*), and so, for the woman who wants to minimize her chance of future surgery, a TAH may be preferable.

The Surgical Approach for Hysterectomy

Most surgeons would agree that if a vaginal hysterectomy can be done, this is the best treatment option. Information suggests that women undergoing vaginal hysterectomy have a quicker recovery and fewer complications than women undergoing an abdominal hysterectomy.[9] Although the approach of vaginal hysterectomy is straightforward with a normal-sized uterus, the larger the fibroids, the more complicated the procedure. Surgeons who are expert with vaginal hysterectomy are often able to remove uteruses that are 12–16 weeks' gestation size; however, it is rare to find a surgeon comfortable with vaginal hysterectomy for a uterus larger than this.

In addition to size, there are other reasons that a vaginal hysterectomy might not be appropriate. If a woman has had prior infection or scar tissue, this would limit the ability to safely remove the uterus without injuring adjacent tissue. For these women, a laparoscopically assisted vaginal hysterectomy may be appropriate. This procedure allows the surgeon to visualize the ovaries and the uterus using a laparoscope placed at the belly button and to be able to potentially perform part of the operation through the small laparoscopic incisions. However, this is generally a more time-consuming and expensive procedure than a regular vaginal hysterectomy. In addition, both of these approaches require removal of the cervix, since the cervix is the first part of the uterus to be freed up in a vaginal approach.

A newer approach is a laparoscopic supracervical hysterectomy. This requires a surgeon with special laparoscopic skills. The upper uterus (fundus) can be mobilized in this way and the cervix left in place. Again, however, size is a factor. If the uterus extends above the belly button, placing a laparoscope in this position to visualize the procedure is difficult. Also, the gynecologist must be able to manipulate the uterus well enough that he or she can go to both the right and the left sides of the uterus to secure the major blood vessels. Sometimes the fibroid extends so far out to the pelvis that this is difficult.

Treatment with a gonadotropin-releasing hormone (GnRH) agonist is sometimes used to facilitate these less invasive treatments,
converting what would have been an abdominal hysterectomy to a
vaginal or laparoscopic approach. However, in addition to considering the side effects (as discussed in Chapter 15) and cost of the medication, before utilizing this option a woman needs to discuss with
her doctor what the odds are that GnRH-agonist treatment will allow
the intended surgery. Although the average uterine shrinkage following several months of GnRH-agonist treatment is 30 to 60 percent,
there is variability, and some women have little or no shrinkage with
therapy. In some situations, given the size and position of the uterus,
75 percent shrinkage might be necessary to make a particular surgical option possible. While in medicine there is no "sure thing," it is
worth knowing at the outset of therapy whether you are aiming for
a long shot or whether you have a good chance of reaching your goal.

As with a laparoscopic myomectomy, with a laparoscopic hysterectomy the tissue needs to be morcellated, or cut into small pieces,
to be removed. Therefore this type of hysterectomy is not appropriate if there is suspicion of cancer. For cancerous tumors, understanding the relationship between the tumor and the other uterine layers
is critical.

Finally, abdominal hysterectomy is usually the last choice for
women with fibroids. But for women with either large fibroids or
prior fibroid surgeries, it is often the only feasible choice. Many of the
considerations regarding the incision, blood loss, and other complications are the same as those discussed in Chapter 10, on abdominal
myomectomies. Complications occurring with hysterectomy appear
to increase with increasing size of the uterus.[10]

Choosing to have a hysterectomy is a difficult decision. In many
ways it was easier in the "good old days," when the doctor made all
the decisions. Most women would like to avoid this major surgery,
however, and it makes good sense to weigh the risk and benefits for
you. However, hysterectomy remains a good choice for women with
large fibroids that are not approachable by other techniques, for
women with prior attempts at symptom control who have had no
success in controlling their symptoms, or for women with recurrent
fibroids.

PART III

Medical Treatment

CHAPTER 14

Traditional Hormonal Therapies: Birth Control Pills and Progestin

When most people think about drugs used for gynecologic purposes, they think first about birth control. High-dose combinations of estrogen and progestin are known as birth control pills (BCPs) or oral contraceptives (OCs). In practice, however, these pills are often also prescribed to provide hormonal therapy for diseases such as fibroids.

Birth control pills have very high levels of both special estrogens and progestins that allow them to be absorbed when taken by mouth. The first generation of OCs had very high hormone levels to prevent ovulation. The BCPs available today have lower hormone levels that often permit ovulation but maintain their contraceptive efficacy through multiple actions such as making the endometrium less hospitable for an embryo and making the cervical mucus thicker and less favorable for sperm transport. Even today's "low-dose" pills have higher doses of steroid hormones than women normally produce in their body.

The chief advantage of oral contraceptives for fibroids is that they control bleeding in some women. It is not clear whether this therapeutic outcome results from controlling the effects of the fibroids or whether the hormones treat a second problem that leads to bleeding, particularly oligoovulation (failure to release an egg).

Estrogen and progestin continuously given together like with OCs lead to a very thin but stable uterine lining. Any thickened endometrium is typically shed within 3 months, which is why most women who have abnormal bleeding see the bleeding resolve within the first three cycles of being on OCs. This is how birth control pills can help decrease the bleeding with fibroids, by thinning the lining.

Many textbooks still state that BCPs should not be used in women with fibroids because of concerns that their fibroids may grow. The high levels of steroid hormones do, in some women, cause the fibroids to grow. However, many women take BCPs for prolonged periods of time and do not seem to experience noticeable fibroid growth. In addition, several studies have suggested that BCPs decrease the chance of fibroids forming.[1-4] However, one of the larger studies suggests that for very young women, age 16 and under, the exposure to OCs may paradoxically increase the risk of fibroids.[1]

Treating women with progesterone or a progestin is also a frequent practice in gynecology. Many progestins are chemically synthesized and have androgen or androgen-like actions (all steroid hormones are similar, and the modification of small parts of the molecule can give a steroid an action similar to that of another, normal hormone). Thus, many progestins are "keys" that fit both the progesterone and androgen "lock."

Progesterone is normally secreted in the time between ovulation and the next period, which is referred to as a luteal or secretory phase. Thus, the side effects of progestins can be similar to those seen in premenstrual syndrome (in which symptoms occur in the luteal phase), with bloating, acne, weight gain, and increased appetite. Progestins can help control bleeding by helping organize endometrium that has been allowed to grow too thick because of oligoovulation.

It is controversial whether progesterone treatment alone is useful for the treatment of fibroids. Because there are so many different formulations of progestins, the type of compound and the way it is used are likely to determine, in part, whether it is effective. Some of the earliest studies done with fibroids suggest that high-dose progesterone would cause the fibroid uterus to shrink. However, those studies were performed in the days before ultrasound, when obtaining objective information was difficult.[5,6]

Several different types of studies have suggested that progesterone may be as important in the control of fibroid growth as estrogen.

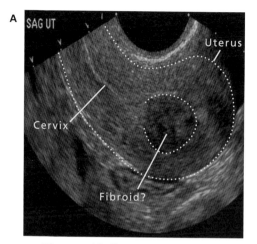

Ultrasound indicating possible fibroid

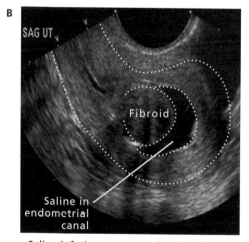

Saline-infusion sonogram showing fibroid

Plate 1. Panel A is a sagittal view of a retroverted uterus (one tipped back toward the woman's spine) obtained by transvaginal ultrasound (TV US). The cervical opening is seen as a narrow white line in the middle left of the image, and the fundus, or top of the uterus, is to the right in each image. Although it appears that there is something dark in the middle of the uterus, it is not well defined on the ultrasound image. Panel B is a saline-infusion sonogram (SIS). With saline (sterile salt water) infused into the endometrial cavity, you can see the fluid filling the top of the cavity (to the right) and outlining the rounded submucosal fibroid that is protruding into the endometrial cavity.

Images courtesy of Dr. Mary Frates, Department of Radiology, Brigham and Women's Hospital and Harvard Medical School, Boston.

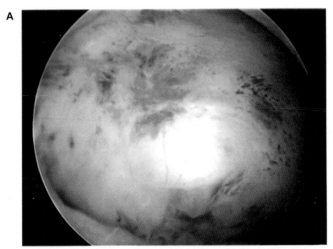

A

Hysteroscopic view of submucosal fibroid

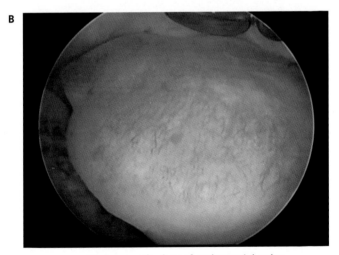

B

Hysteroscopic view of endometrial polyp

Plate 2. A pair of photographs taken during a hysteroscopy. Both lesions are large and fill the endometrial cavity. Panel A shows a submucosal fibroid. Submucosal fibroids are typically whiter and appear shinier because of the increased amount of extracellular matrix. They also often have bigger blood vessels or a coarser pattern of vessels. Panel B shows a polyp. A polyp tends to have softer edges, and at times you can even see little areas of what appear to be gland openings like pinpricks across the surface. Polyps also sometimes have filmy cotton-candy-type adhesions holding them to the endometrium.

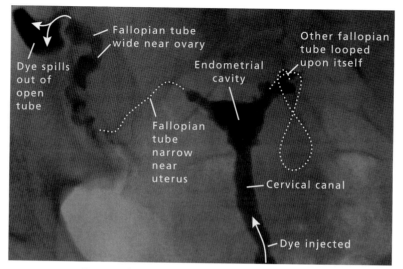

Dye spills
out of
open
tube

Fallopian tube
wide near ovary

Other fallopian
tube looped
upon itself

Endometrial
cavity

Fallopian
tube
narrow
near
uterus

Cervical canal

Dye injected

Hysterosalpingogram visualizing fallopian tube

Plate 3. The woman whose hysterosalpingogram (HSG) is shown here had previous surgery for uterine fibroids. In an HSG, an iodine-containing "dye" is injected into the uterus and fallopian tubes through the cervix, and X-rays are used to take the pictures. You cannot see the wall of the uterus or the ovaries, but an HSG is the best test for seeing the fallopian tubes. In this image the uterus is the triangular-shaped area to the right of the center. It is somewhat irregular because of the previous myomectomy or new small fibroids. The cervix, which is below the uterus, is very long. The fallopian tube on the left side of the picture is spread out so that you can see that it begins as a very thin line; the opening gets larger as it approaches the open end. At the left top corner is a "blob" of dye that has come out of the fallopian tube and pooled around the bowel, indicating that the tube is open. The other fallopian tube is also open, though we cannot see this clearly in this image.

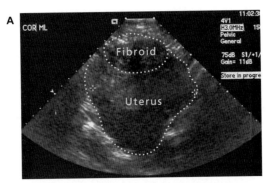

Pelvic ultrasound of uterine fibroid

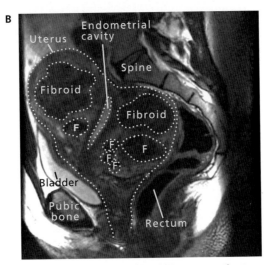

Pelvic MRI of uterine fibroid in same patient

Plate 4. These two images illustrate the difference between a pelvic ultrasound (Panel A) and a pelvic MRI (Panel B). Both are of the same uterus taken several weeks apart. Although the ultrasound image captures the basic information about size of the uterus and the presence or absence of a fibroid, the MRI can provide more detail. In this T2 weighted MRI, the dark oval in the lower left-hand corner is the pubic bone, and the white crescent-shaped area above that is the bladder, which is stretched out by the fibroid uterus. The whitish area perpendicular to the bladder is the endometrial cavity. In this sagittal view, you see one big fibroid and one smaller fibroid in front of the endometrial cavity and several smaller fibroids behind it. You can also see that the fibroid uterus reaches all the way back to the curvature of the spine, which could cause back pain. The sacrum is also visible. The bowel is behind the uterus, and you can see that there may be some compression of the bowel as well.

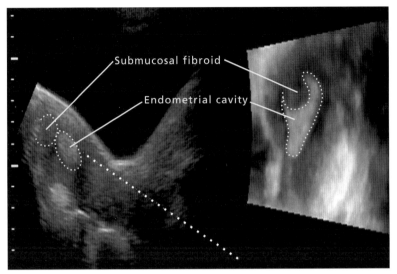

Three-dimensional ultrasound of submucosal fibroid

Plate 5. Three-dimensional (3D) ultrasound can give better definition to structures in the endometrial cavity. On the left is a transvaginal ultrasound scan, in which it is clear there is a mass in the endometrial cavity (the white area), but the extent of protrusion into the cavity is not clear. The dotted line shows the plane of the 3D ultrasound image acquisition, which is pictured in the insertion on the right side of the image. In the 3D image it is clear this is a Type I submucosal fibroid arising from the uterine fundus and therefore able to be treated with hysteroscopic myomectomy.

Images courtesy of Dr. Faye Laing, Professor of Radiology, Brigham and Women's Hospital and Harvard Medical School, Boston.

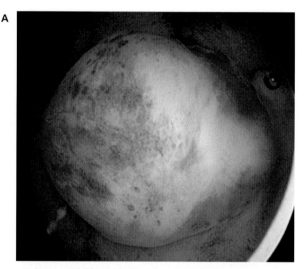

A

Submucosal fibroid before hysteroscopic myomectomy

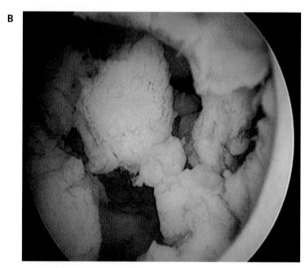

B

Fragments of resected fibroid before removal

Plate 6. The submucosal fibroid is seen in Panel A at the beginning of a hysteroscopic myomectomy. In Panel B, multiple fragments of fibroid resected by the resectoscope are floating within the cavity before being removed through the cervix.

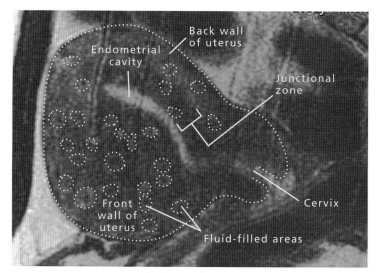

T2 weighted MRI of adenomyosis

Plate 7. On this T2 weighted MRI scan, adenomyosis is indicated by the appearance of white areas in the normally dark myometrium as well as by thickening of the junctional zone, the darker stripe between the endometrium and the myometrium. In this image, the front wall of the uterus is more than twice as thick as the posterior wall as a result of adenomyosis.

First, people have always correlated the states in which estrogen levels are high (e.g., pregnancy) with fibroid growth and states in which estrogen levels are low (e.g., menopause and following treatment with a gonadotropin-releasing hormone [GnRH] agonist) with fibroid shrinkage. This correlation has been extended to argue that estrogen is the important influence on fibroid behavior. However, progesterone levels generally follow estrogen levels in these states, so that progesterone is high during pregnancy and low following menopause and GnRH-agonist therapy.

Second, when GnRH agonists were first being used, the thought was that they could be combined with progestin treatment to provide some support for the woman's bone density and protection against hot flashes and not cause regrowth of fibroids. However, studies then performed suggested that fibroids failed to shrink when progestin was administered with a GnRH agonist.[7,8]

More recently, drugs whose primary mechanism of action is to block the action of progestins have been shown to be effective in decreasing fibroid symptoms. The most widely studied is the drug mifepristone (discussed in more detail in Chapter 16).[9–11] Nonetheless, there are studies that suggest that women getting continuous progestin exposure for contraception (such as Depo-Provera) may actually have a decreased risk of fibroid formation.[2] This has recently been confirmed in a large study of African American women. Finally, the use of Mirena, a progestin-containing intrauterine device (IUD), has been shown to substantially decrease bleeding in women with normal uteruses and women with fibroids.[12–14]

One of the issues that is not clear is whether the composition of the steroid hormones is the most important factor, or whether maintaining an acyclic environment (not having monthly menses) is what is important. In the normal menstrual cycle, the levels of estrogen and progesterone are actively changing at many points during the cycle. Oral contraceptive pills, particularly monophasic pills (meaning that every tablet contains the same composition of drug), keep the steroid hormone environment constant. Some people have hypothesized that this constant environment is one of the benefits of pregnancy. Even though the steroid hormone levels are high during pregnancy, they stay high throughout pregnancy and don't have the constant monthly changes that occur when women are having regular menstrual cycles. Thus, although pregnancy, with high hormone levels, and GnRH-agonist treatment, with low hormone levels, initially seem to be at opposite ends of the hormonal spectrum, both can treat gynecologic diseases including fibroids because there is no constant hormonal cycling.

As noted earlier, I like to think about the acyclic environment very much like turning on and off a light bulb. If you keep flicking the switch back and forth rapidly, you are more likely to have a blown light bulb than if you keep it on and leave it on for hours, if not days. Thus, part of the problem with fibroids may be the constant switching back and forth. A stable environment may be the reason that all the different hormone environments (very low estrogen plus progesterone, high estrogen plus progesterone, and progesterone-dominant) work to decrease symptoms.

CHAPTER 15

GnRH Agonists, Add-Back Therapies, and GnRH Antagonists

GnRH Agonists

Gonadotropin-releasing hormone (GnRH) agonists have been the mainstay of medical treatment for uterine fibroids. As discussed in Chapter 4, the hourly pulses of the brain hormone GnRH are critical to normal reproductive function; without GnRH, the ovaries and uterus return to the state they were in before puberty. Interfering with the GnRH system shuts down the entire reproductive system, and this mechanism can be used to treat uterine fibroids.

GnRH agonists are the major class of drugs used in the treatment of fibroids and other gynecologic diseases, including endometriosis and polycystic ovaries. An agonist is a substance that acts like the hormone in question. Therefore, GnRH agonists (a key) bind to GnRH receptors (the lock) and act just like GnRH. The difference between GnRH and GnRH agonists is that the latter molecules have been engineered so that the body does not break them down quite as rapidly. Therefore, they are like long-acting GnRH, and their effect on the body is like having natural GnRH around for long periods of time without the critical pulses.

Thus, when a woman takes a GnRH agonist, luteinizing hormone (LH) and follicle-stimulating hormone (FSH) are initially stimulated,

which leads to stimulation of estrogen and, in some cases, progesterone, which can lead to a "flare" in symptoms, especially bleeding.
Fairly soon after, however, the system shuts down and the levels of
LH, FSH, estrogen, and progesterone decrease to the levels that exist
before puberty (the down-regulated phase). This is how GnRH agonists function to treat uterine fibroids.

This low-estrogen, low-progesterone state is often incorrectly
termed a medical menopause. In menopause the levels of FSH and
LH are high, whereas following GnRH-agonist treatment these hormone levels are low. We know that in most women menopause leads
to shrinkage of the uterus and no menstrual periods. Therefore, the
terminology is useful for indicating what happens, even though it
may not accurately describe the hormonal patterns. The first report
of using GnRH agonist to treat fibroids was in 1983, and there have
been numerous studies since that time.[1-2] Most women have a reduction in uterine volume between 30 and 60 percent with 3 to 6
months of therapy. Both the fibroid and the normal myometrium
undergo shrinkage.[3] Most women will also stop having periods,
although some women will have a heavy bleed as the estrogen levels
climb during the first, or flare, phase.

Considering this good response, why aren't GnRH agonists more
widely used for the treatment of fibroids? There are several reasons.
First, these medications have significant side effects; for this reason,
women do not want to take them for long periods. The side effects are
exaggerated symptoms of menopause, including hot flashes, difficulty
sleeping, muscle aches or pain, and changes in concentration and
mood. Just as young women whose ovaries are surgically removed can
often have more severe menopause symptoms than a woman who has
been gradually transitioning over a number of years, side effects of
GnRH-agonist treatment can be severe for some women.

Second, even if a woman tolerates these low-estrogen side effects,
bone tissue cannot stay strong without estrogen. Like menopausal
women, women undergoing long-term GnRH-agonist treatment tend
to have accelerated bone loss that can lead to osteoporosis. Therefore,
treatment is usually restricted to 6 months or less, or the bone density is actively monitored.

Third, there is no carryover effect. After GnRH-agonist treatment
is stopped, there is a rapid return of symptoms and a rebound of the
uterus to its original size, or sometimes bigger. Therefore, unlike some

medications, a short-term treatment will not give long-term results. Finally, the expense and inconvenience of long-term medical therapy limit its use.

For all these reasons, although GnRH agonists are very effective medications, they are used now only in preparation for surgery, as a temporizing agent for women with acute medical issues, or for women who are close to menopause.

Many formulations of GnRH agonist are available worldwide. The earliest forms of GnRH agonist were given as daily injections. Daily shots are almost never used for the treatment of fibroids, although they are still widely used as a part of infertility treatments. The daily treatment that is still used for fibroids is the nasal spray Synarel. Most women, however, use a long-acting form of the drug. In the United States, Lupron is available as both a 1-month and a 3-month Depo injection, and Zoladex is a 1-month and a 3-month injectable implant. The only medical therapy for fibroids approved by the Food and Drug Administration (FDA) involves the use of the GnRH agonist Lupron for the presurgical treatment of uterine fibroids to correct anemia in conjunction with iron administration (see Chapter 10, on abdominal myomectomy).

Add-Back Therapies

Many strategies have been tried to extend the use of GnRH agonists to provide women with longer-term relief. These strategies are termed the *add-back therapies*. Additional drugs are *added back* to the GnRH agonist to give some relief of the hypoestrogenic (low-estrogen) symptoms without raising the level of hormones to the point where the fibroids regrow. The traditional add-backs have been low doses of estrogen or progestin (or both). It is important when evaluating the steroidal add-back regimens to pay attention to both *the kind* of hormone given and *how* it is given relative to the GnRH agonist.

The two most widely tested regimens involve adding back either medroxyprogesterone acetate (a synthetic progestin used widely in hormone therapy) or estrogen plus progestin combinations used in menopausal hormone therapy.[4–6]

Originally it was thought that since estrogen was the important hormone for fibroids, simply using a progestin would be the perfect add-back. However, two early studies found that although women's periods stopped with this regimen, the uterus did not shrink. This was the first time physicians began to wonder whether progestins played an important role in fibroids.

How the GnRH agonist is given in relationship to the add-back can also be important with steroid hormones. Add-back can be started at the same time as the GnRH agonist (this is called *simultaneous administration*), or the GnRH agonist can be started first; in that case, only after the low-estrogen or down-regulated state is reached are the steroid hormones added back (*sequential administration*), since these two steps happen in sequence.[2] For many disease processes, such as endometriosis and abnormal hair growth (hirsutism), simultaneous add-backs have been successful. To produce uterine shrinkage with fibroids, however, a sequential regimen, with progestin or estrogen-progestin regimens, is preferable.

The other important point regarding steroid hormone add-backs for fibroids is that they need to be low dose, such as those used for postmenopausal hormone replacement, rather than high dose, as in birth control pills. Although birth control add-back can work for diseases such as hirsutism, a lower level of steroid hormones is necessary for the treatment of fibroids. There are also preliminary results suggesting that using low-dose estradiol alone in a simultaneous add-back regimen can be potentially useful.[7]

Some studies are exploring the use of innovative steroidal compounds for add-back therapies. The selective estrogen receptor modulators (SERMs) tamoxifen and raloxifene both appear to be very effective treatments for fibroids in animals.[8] However, in several small studies of humans, standard doses of SERMs have not been effective with GnRH agonists for the treatment of fibroids, although one study of a very high dose SERM showed some benefit.[9,10]

Tibolone is used outside the United States as a single-agent medical therapy for hormone replacement, since it has both estrogen- and progesterone-like actions.[11] It appears to result in less vaginal bleeding than ordinary estrogen-progestin hormone therapy both in the general postmenopausal population and specifically in women with uterine fibroids.[11,12] Ipriflavone, which is a weak estrogen, and isoflavone (a phytoestrogen, one derived from plants, and an antioxidant) have also been used in women participating in a small study, with good results.[13] In addition, researchers have experimented with adding compounds such as calcium to make strong bones.

GnRH Antagonists

GnRH antagonists are also effective treatments for uterine fibroids. These drugs bind to the GnRH receptor and lead the system to shut down without the flare effect seen with GnRH agonists. The first GnRH antagonists tended to have significant side effects, which made GnRH agonists better treatment options. However, several different formulations have been shown to provide effective treatment for uterine fibroids.[14–16] In addition to having no flare, the antagonists work more quickly (over days to weeks rather than months) to bring levels of estrogen and progesterone down to menopausal levels.

GnRH antagonists are available in the United States, since they are FDA-approved for use in ovarian stimulation for women in in vitro fertilization (IVF) fertility procedures. However, the doses available for IVF are different from those tested with fibroids, and because the medications are packaged for use for only a few days at a time, they are difficult to use in treating fibroids.

CHAPTER 16

Innovative Medical Strategies for Treating Uterine Fibroids

Innovative Steroidal Therapies

Medical therapies that manipulate either estrogen or progesterone in an innovative way have been used for fibroid therapy. The most extensively studied is the progesterone-modulating drug mifepristone. Early studies used relatively high doses (25–50 mg a day) for relatively short exposures (up to several months).[1-3] In these studies, mifepristone, like GnRH agonists, was very effective in the treatment of uterine fibroids and stopped menstrual periods in almost all women and caused substantial fibroid shrinkage of 30–60 percent. The major advantage of mifepristone over GnRH agonists is that with mifepristone treatment women maintained a low to normal level of estrogen. Thus, women had fewer symptoms such as hot flashes and should have high enough estrogen levels to maintain bone density.

The most troubling finding with mifepristone is that the endometrium had specific changes; the changes were not precancerous but were nonetheless worrisome.[3] This concern stems from our understanding that progesterone is the major brake on the progression of chronically estrogen-exposed endometrium to precancerous changes and cancer. Therefore drugs that block progesterone may make a woman more susceptible to this endometrial cancer. Subsequent studies with a lower dose (5 mg) suggest that these previously seen endometrial changes may be due to the higher dose and that relatively good control of fibroid symptoms can be achieved with lower doses.[4,5] There was also concern with the higher doses (but not the lower doses) that mifepristone might interfere with the action of another class of important steroid hormones, the glucocorticoids, including the important stress hormone cortisol.[1]

Although mifepristone is available in the United States, as with GnRH antagonists, the marketed doses make it difficult to provide effective treatment for uterine fibroids. The single marketed dose is 600 mg; to divide this dose into any of the previously tested doses of mifepristone requires a compounding pharmacy to make a specific formulation.

A newer generation of more selective progesterone-modulating compounds is under development; they are often termed *progesterone receptor modulators* (PRMs) or *selective progesterone receptor modulators* (SPRMs). The compound Asoprisnil (previously referred to as J867) has been used in clinical trials for uterine fibroids, but only preliminary information is available about its efficacy.[6,7] Additional PRMs are undergoing testing for the treatment of uterine fibroids, but results have not yet been reported in the scientific literature.

Although estrogen-modulating compounds have shown great effectiveness in animal models of fibroids, the results to date in women have been disappointing.[8] The SERM raloxifene has been shown in small studies to be effective in treating postmenopausal women with fibroids and as a GnRH-agonist add-back regimen.[9,10] Initial studies in premenopausal women with the standard dose of raloxifene used for menopausal hormone therapy showed no effectiveness; use of 3 times this standard dose did not cause fibroid or uterine shrinkage but did keep the fibroids from increasing in size over 3 months.[11] This small benefit will have to be weighed against the risk of complications, since even the standard dose of raloxifene is associated with an increased risk of blood clots, or thrombosis.

Finally, targeting the enzyme aromatase (which converts androgens to estrogens) may be an important therapy of the future. Aromatase inhibitors (blockers) are used in the treatment of hormonally responsive cancers, and scientific studies suggest they may be helpful in the treatment of gynecologic disease like endometriosis and fibroids.[12]

Nonsteroidal Hormonal Therapies

All the drugs we currently use to treat fibroids manipulate estrogen or progesterone to achieve a therapeutic effect. This approach is based on the research showing that fibroids were different in biologic ways from normal myometrium: they had more receptors for estrogen or progesterone (or both), and they were more sensitive to potent estrogens and progestins. Understanding new elements of fibroid biology will likely lead to new treatments that approach fibroids in different ways. For example, if you start to think about fibroids as a disease of fibrosis or scar tissue rather than as a disease of steroid hormones, whole new targets for therapy develop. Although none of these treatments has been approved by the FDA yet, it is likely that these new treatment options will develop over the next decade.

Similar patterns have been seen in other diseases. Ulcer disease was once thought to be related only to stomach acid production. However, there is now good evidence that particular bacteria living in the stomach contribute to this disease process, so some ulcers can be treated with antibiotics and Pepto-Bismol. There are several hints that other biologic systems may be able to be manipulated to produce improvement in fibroid symptoms.

As we discussed earlier, the angiogenic growth factor called basic fibroblast growth factor (bFGF) appears to be important in the biology of fibroids. Interferon-α (alpha) and interferon-β (beta) are compounds that are known to interfere with bFGF in other biological systems. There was an unusual report from Japan of a woman who was treated with interferon-α for a totally separate disease (hepatitis-C). The doctors taking care of her noted that she had a very large fibroid prior to starting the therapy and that, after seventeen months of therapy, the fibroid had shrunk to approximately one-tenth its previous volume.[13] The most interesting finding was that after only a short treatment with interferon the fibroid remained small for more than a year and a half. This is particularly interesting because interferons usually have a carryover effect; when used for the treatment of multiple sclerosis, a 6-month treatment can produce improvement of symptoms for more than a year.

A single report like this does not mean that the interferon was necessarily the cause of this change. For example, the interferon could have improved liver functions so that estrogen was processed differently. However, the results are striking enough that trying this type of therapy in women with fibroids may be useful.

Also, small studies from Italy suggest that interfering with the insulin-like growth factor (IGF) and growth hormone (GH) systems may be appropriate treatment for women with fibroids. Using a drug called lanoreotide for 3 months caused a reduction in uterine volume of approximately 24 percent; again, there were some carryover effects.[14] Lanoreotide is a somatostatin-like drug (somatostatin is a natural hormone produced in the body) that is used to treat an excessive growth hormone disorder called acromegaly. It has orphan drug status in the United States and is not widely available. (An orphan drug is a drug developed under a 1983 act of Congress making it possible for drug companies to receive a tax reduction for developing drugs to treat rare diseases.)

Drugs that target fibrosis or fibrotic factors might also be useful in the treatment of fibroids.[15,16] Compounds that have been tested in laboratory experiments include pirfenidone and halofuginone.[17]

Signaling molecules, the molecules that transmit directions to the cell after a protein hormone binds to the cell surface (as we discussed in Chapter 4), may also provide novel targets. Again, one particular molecule, peroxisome proliferator-activated receptor gamma (PPAR-γ) has been tested in laboratory experiments.[18]

Gene therapy may also be an avenue for future treatments. Laboratory experiments suggest that cell-to-cell communication is so strong in fibroids that only a small percentage of cells need to be targeted to lead to substantial cell death with gene therapy.[19]

PART IV

Other Factors, Other Conditions

CHAPTER 17

The Genetics of Fibroids

It is hard to explain why the genetics of fibroids is so important when we currently know so little about it. However, from studies in other fields, it is increasingly clear that the genes people are born with cause them to be at risk for certain diseases. The genes are really the instructions for all the body-building parts, and they can cause malfunctions in the same manner that the instructions and materials used in building a car can make some cars prone to brake failures and others prone to engine overheating. We begin life with instructions that program our body to respond in particular ways. Beginning with this assumption, we believe that genes influence a woman's ability to develop fibroids and also probably influence whether they cause bleeding, increase in size, or are quick to form again after surgery.

The discovery of the structure of DNA (deoxyribonucleic acid) by Watson and Crick revolutionized biology and medicine.[1] They discovered that DNA carries the code for life in a ladderlike structure. The ladder is twisted to form a "double helix" and then packaged with proteins so it can fit into the nucleus of the cell in bundles termed *chromosomes*. The rungs of the ladder are the important part; each rung has a pair of molecules—either an adenosine and a thymine (AT or TA pair) or a guanine and a cytosine (GC or CG pair)— that have molecular attraction for each other so that they are held together as if they were held with a magnet. Not only do other pairings not have that attractive force, but a GA or AG pair would be too big to fit in the ladder and a TC or CT pair too small.

The beauty of the ladder-helix structure is that when it comes time to make a new cell and the rungs of the ladder come apart (since they are held by magnetic attraction and not joined solidly together), each half contains all the information needed to make two complete copies. The chromosome half with a G knows to pair with a C, and the opposite strand with a C pairs automatically with a G. The two strands are thus called complementary. With this elegant mechanism information is passed not only from one cell to another but on to the next generation.[2]

The genes are coded in long strings of As, Ts, Gs, and Cs in the DNA of the nucleus of a cell. They are translated into working code called RNA. This RNA leaves the nucleus and goes out into the cytoplasm, where the cell's factory manufactures all the body's protein. I will sometimes refer to the DNA and the protein by the same name, but the DNA is really the direction for making the working protein.

Genotype and Phenotype

Before going further, it is important to define the terms *genotype* and *phenotype*. The genotype is the pattern of genes that you inherit. For example, with eye color, brown is a dominant color and is represented by a "B." Blue is a recessive trait and represented by a "b." Therefore, a person can have "BB," "bb," or "Bb" as genotypes for eye color. Each person gets two copies of the gene, one originally from his or her mother and the other from his or her father. The dominant gene will always dominate; it has the power to trump a recessive trait. (See fig. 17.1.)

Phenotype is the physical manifestation, or end result, of the genotype. Although there are three different genotypes (BB, bb, or Bb), there are only two phenotypes: brown eyes and blue eyes. People with the "BB" or the "Bb" genotype have brown eyes because brown is the dominant trait; only the people with the "bb" genotype have blue eyes. (See fig. 17.2.)

Genotype, Phenotype, and Fibroids

I believe that fibroids are a common phenotype that represents many different underlying genotypes. In other words, in my view, fibroids

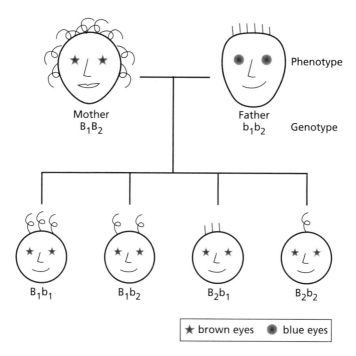

All four children have different genotypes, but the same phenotype brown eyes.

Figure 17.1. In this example regarding eye color, the mother has two dominant genes and has brown eyes, while the father has two recessive genes and has blue eyes. Since each child will receive a dominant gene from his or her mother, all the children will have brown eyes (the same phenotype, or appearance), even though each one has a different genotype (combination of Bs and bs). If the gene carried the risk for fibroids, all the daughters would have fibroids, and the sons would pass the risk on to approximately half of their daughters.

can arise through multiple different pathways. In this case, "Bb" might represent two different genes that code for the estrogen receptor beta, which influences the action of estrogen on fibroid tissue. A "B" may make the fibroid more sensitive to this hormone and therefore more likely to grow. In addition, probably multiple genes influence fibroids, so that in addition to "Bb" we may also have "Pp" for progesterone receptors, "Ff" for fibrotic factors, and so on.

It is also likely that with further study we will be able to refine the phenotype of fibroids. Consider what has happened over the past century with cancer. Originally any uncontrolled growth was called,

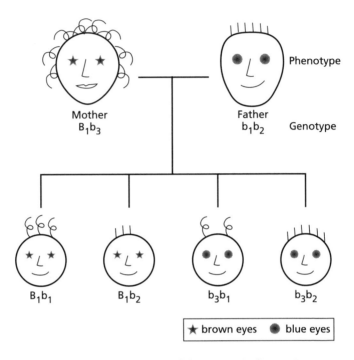

With the same phenotypes of the parents in figure 17.1,
the children have different phenotypes.

Figure 17.2. In this case, although the parents have the same phenotype as in the previous example (the mother has brown eyes and the father has blue eyes), the mother is heterozygous. This means she has one gene for blue eyes and one for brown eyes, but because brown is dominant, it trumps the recessive gene. However, in this case, half of the children will have blue eyes because they have only recessive genes and can express the phenotype of blue eyes.

simply, cancer. With further study it became evident that different tissues in the body formed different kinds of cancers. Finally, over the past few decades, we have been able to pinpoint certain molecules that cause certain cancers. Therefore, we have identified not only leukemia but also acute lymphocytic leukemia (ALL), acute myelogenous leukemia (AML), and so on. A diversity of phenotypes may explain the diversity of symptoms that we see with fibroids. Eventually we may be able to explain why some women have heavy bleeding but never develop large fibroids and why other women have large fibroids but never have bleeding problems.

A definition of further types of fibroids based on genotype may be useful in determining prognosis. A prognosis means predicting, in advance, the likelihood of problems and outcomes with the disease. For example, a fibroid that has a bad prognosis may be one that reappears and requires surgery within 2 years of the original myomectomy. Knowing that this was a "bad prognosis fibroid" may be helpful in counseling particular women as they face treatment decisions. Knowing this information prior to or shortly after a myomectomy, for example, may encourage a woman who is thinking about future pregnancy to have a pregnancy sooner rather than later.

This information would be most helpful in advance of treatment, so that the woman who carried a high risk of recurrent fibroids and had completed her family might even choose to have a hysterectomy because her chance of having an additional surgery was so high. We currently have some clinical information (based on physicians' clinical experience with many patients) to predict prognosis for recurrence after abdominal myomectomy, but our clinical information for any other kind of treatment options is limited.

Finally, understanding the underlying genotype would open up important possibilities for the future. It may, for example, point to ways in which women can modify their risk of disease and lead to prevention of disease. If, for example, a major protein involved in body fat metabolism was found to be abnormally sensitive in women with fibroids, weight loss or preventing weight gain might be an effective strategy for decreasing the risk of fibroids. In this day and age, new therapies can be developed that are targeted to specific abnormalities; this is what happened with chronic myelogenous leukemia (CML) and Gleevec, which combats this disease with minimal side effects.

Evidence for the Role of Genes in Fibroid Development and Growth

Studies of women with fibroids suggest several reasons to suspect that genes play a role in fibroid formation. The first is that both women in a pair of identical twins are twice as likely to have had a hysterectomy as both women in a pair of fraternal (nonidentical) twins. Identical twins share 100 percent of their genes, while fraternal twins share only 50 percent of their genes. This suggests that the genes that identical twins share make them more likely to form fibroids, since both identical and nonidentical twins have equal exposure to environmental factors. This difference between identical and fraternal twins has been observed in a general population of women undergoing hysterectomy and a population of women with fibroids leading to hysterectomy.[3,4]

There is also evidence that women who have close relatives, such as a mother or sister, with fibroids are much more likely to have fibroids themselves.[5,6] This propensity is called *familial aggregation*. Just as with breast cancer, if you have many relatives affected by fibroids, your risk of disease is likely to be increased.

Some women appear to inherit an increased risk from their father and not their mother. In these women, none of their maternal relatives has fibroids, but all their paternal aunts and cousins have fibroids. This connection raises the intriguing question of what a "fibroid gene" causes in the men who have it.

In addition, in some rare syndromes fibroids are found clustered with other disorders. The repeated clustering of three or four rare problems suggests that the clustering does not occur by chance and that there is a single gene linking all these unusual problems.

Hereditary leiomyomatosis and renal cell carcinoma (HLRCC) syndrome is one such rare but important syndrome involving fibroids.[7,8] In families with HLRCC syndrome, not only do women have fibroids, but both men and women in the family have fibroid-like lesions in the skin (cutaneous leiomyomas). These skin lesions can be so small that they are difficult to see, but they can be felt under the skin, similar to "goose bumps" that never go away. Alternatively, they can be the size and texture of a mosquito bite.

Individuals with the gene that leads to both fibroids and skin leiomyomas are also at an increased risk for a rare type of kidney cell cancer (papillary renal cell carcinoma, or RCC); for reasons we do not know, women in these families develop this kidney cancer more often than men. These women are also more likely to develop uterine sarcomas (cancerous tumors of the uterus).

Just as we search for the rare families with the breast cancer genes BRCA 1 and BRCA 2, to lead to early diagnosis of cancer, we need to search for HLRCC syndrome. The key to this search is to look for the cutaneous leiomyomas. We are able to reassure most women that fibroids are benign tumors and that they are exceedingly unlikely to have a cancerous sarcoma. However, if you have the gene for HLRCC syndrome, you are at increased risk for cancer, both in the uterus (sarcoma) and in the kidney (RCC). Since the HLRCC syndrome is inherited in a dominant fashion, most people who have the gene will have the skin lesions. It does not skip generations, so grandparents, parents, and some children may all have the syndrome.

There is a test for the HLRCC syndrome gene, but it is not yet widely available. If the genetic testing is not performed in your area, by enrolling in a study through the National Institutes of Health, families can be tested (http://clinicalstudies.info.nih.gov, protocol 03-C-0066). Testing for the gene causing the syndrome is important because it can identify people at risk for cancer early, and in some cases the cancer can be prevented. Gene testing can also identify family members who do not have the gene and thus have no increased risk.

Both of the cancers associated with HLRCC syndrome are atypical. The kidney cancer has an unusual microscopic pattern called papillary renal cell carcinoma, and it behaves very aggressively. Often it has metastasized (spread throughout the body) by the time it is diagnosed. This is why screening needs to be undertaken in people at risk, to catch the cancer early or prevent it.

Sarcomas, or uterine cancers, usually develop in women after menopause (see Chapter 20), but in women with HLRCC syndrome, sarcomas develop in younger, premenopausal women. For women with symptomatic fibroids who have HLRCC syndrome, hysterectomy may be the best choice to decrease or eliminate the risk of cancer.[9]

There are two other names for HLRCC syndrome: Reed's syndrome and multiple cutaneous and uterine leiomyomas (MCUL1) syndrome.[10] Although many textbooks describe these three as different syndromes, because we have learned that the same gene causes all three, the older names will likely disappear.

Other rare syndromes that involve fibroids and other benign skin lesions include Bannayan-Zonana syndrome.[11] In this syndrome, again, both women and men may have skin lipomas (fatty skin tumors) or hemangiomas (blood-vessel-filled tumors). The gene for this syndrome is also a dominant gene, so it is likely that someone in each generation has the gene and thus the skin lesions.

Information about genetic syndromes can be found through a Web site created by the Johns Hopkins School of Medicine called OMIM:

Online Mendelian Inheritance in Man (www3.ncbi.nlm.nih.gov/ entrez/query.fcgi?db=OMIM). Gregor Mendel is the monk who first described genes as the packet of information that codes for different traits in pea plants. Thus, *Mendelian*, a term that refers to traits inherited by genes, is used in honor of Mendel.

Molecular Genetics

Understanding which genes are involved in fibroids doesn't automatically tell us why fibroids develop or how to control them. From our understanding of fibroid behavior, we would guess that genes involved in estrogen or progesterone production, metabolism, or action would be involved. Unfortunately, science is seldom that straightforward. Most guesses regarding these "candidate genes" turn out to be wrong, and much study is usually required to find out how these genes lead to disease.

The hunt for genes involved in fibroid formation starts with finding chromosomes that are broken in characteristic places in fibroids just like the Philadelphia chromosome was linked with CML (discussed in Chapter 3). If a particular abnormal chromosome pattern is associated with fibroids, it suggests that a gene near this point in the chromosome is playing an important role in producing fibroids.[12,13]

Furthermore, the pattern of the broken chromosome provides a clue to how a gene is working to cause fibroids. If parts of two different genes are stuck together, as is the case with the Philadelphia chromosome (a translocation), one of two things may occur: if the break occurs in the middle of the code for the gene, a new (fusion) protein is created; if the break occurs outside the gene (the regulatory region), the instructions for turning the gene on or off may be changed. Thus, a particular gene that is supposed to be turned off in adults may, as a result of a break in the regulatory region, get maximally turned on instead. If a part of the chromosome is missing (deletion), then something that normally puts the brakes on for normal myometrium (tumor suppressor) is lost; if an extra part of the chromosome is present, it may produce an extra copy of a protein that leads to fibroids.

One gene in particular was identified through this method where there was a translocation between chromosomes 12 and 14. The name of this gene is *HMGA2* (also called *HMG I*-C).[14] The HMG part of the name stands for "high mobility group" and is a protein that is highly mobile and goes into the nucleus of the cell to turn on DNA. *HMGA2* appears to be involved in body fat metabolism. Mice that have an abnormality of the related gene have small amounts of body fat.[15] It is not yet clear how an abnormal *HMGA2* gene leads to fibroids. We would not have predicted that a "fibroid gene" made a small mouse with less fat; we would have intuitively imagined a big fibrotic mouse would result.

Likewise, the abnormal gene causing both MCUL1 and HLRCC syndrome was a surprise. The responsible gene was identified by studying large family groups (cohorts) with disease. One research group was following a family affected by MCUL1, and the other was studying HLRCC families. They both found the same gene on chromosome 1, *fumarate hydratase* (*FH*), linked to the clinical findings of the syndrome.[7,16]

The *FH* gene codes for a protein that is a part of the Krebs cycle, a group of enzymes active in every cell that allows the body to extract energy from molecules. Again, it is not directly clear why this protein would lead to fibroids. However, some recent studies suggest that it may have something to do with fibroid cells being deprived of oxygen (hypoxia) and leading to new blood vessel formation (angiogenesis).[17] This theory argues that fibroids may result as a response to injury during menstruation, as discussed in Chapter 5.[18]

However, the mutations in the *FH* gene causing HLRCC syndrome lead to nonworking or absent *FH* protein.[8,16] We say that *FH* works as a tumor suppressor gene: normal *FH* suppresses the formation of these tumors, and only when it is inactivated by mutations does a problem arise. Another tumor suppressor gene, phosphatase and tensin homolog (*PTEN*), appears to cause Bannayan-Zonana syndrome, discussed earlier.[11] Loss of tumor suppressor genes is a common process in the formation of cancerous tumors as well as benign tumors such as fibroids.

One explanation for the prevalence of fibroids may be that tumor suppressor genes play a vital role in fibroid formation. The process begins like a car sitting at the top of a hill in neutral gear. You don't have to depress the car's accelerator to start going downhill—you just have to let your foot slip off the brake. If the tumor suppressor is gone, all or most women will form fibroids just as all or most cars in neutral gear with no brakes will roll downhill.

Why would nature want a gene for fibroids to be passed on to new generations of women? It is likely that fibroids are a by-product of some other important process. The genes that lead to fibroid formation probably provide some benefit, just as the mutations that produce sickle cell anemia protect people against malaria. Perhaps the gene had a role in uterine smooth muscle cells that made the uterus contract better following delivery, so that women had less bleeding following delivery. Or it could have had a role in a completely different part of the body, like making a change in the intestine to protect against parasites that could cause diarrhea.

Does *FH* play a role in women with fibroids who have no evidence of the cutaneous leiomyomas? In a small number of women it does. This has been seen in a group of women in Finland and in the United States.[19,20] In the U.S. cohort, *FH* was seen to play a role only in Caucasian women and not at all in black women. This finding underscores the importance of doing studies of fibroids in a racially diverse group, since different genes may be important in different racial groups.

There are also small variations called polymorphisms in genes that may play a role in influencing the risk of fibroids. Both polymorphisms and mutations are changes in the sequence of genes, but the difference is in the degree of change. A mutation makes a major change in the gene that leads to a change in the protein the gene is coding for. It changes the amino acid from alanine to glycine, for example, or causes the protein to be prematurely cut off.

A polymorphism produces a more subtle change. It may change the DNA but keep the protein the same, or it may be outside the gene in the regulatory region so that the gene is more easily turned on or off. There have been some reports of polymorphism of particular steroid-hormone-related genes that appear to increase a woman's risk of developing fibroids.[21–24]

A number of experiments have also been conducted with gene chips (see Chapter 3) to find whole series of genes that are turned off or on in fibroids compared with normal myometrium.[25–27] Just as in cancer, there is probably not one master switch involved in fibroid formation. Instead, a series of genetic changes are likely responsible for fibroid formation, fibroid growth, and the production of symptoms.

Genome-Wide Scan for Fibroid Genes

Finally, in the age of molecular genetics, we can look for genes involved in a disease which are not marked by chromosome breaks, effectively looking for a needle in a haystack. This process is called a *genome-wide scan*. This is a common approach to finding genes in complex diseases, such as diabetes, asthma, and heart disease. With a genome-wide scan women who are sisters and both have fibroids (an affected sibling pair) are recruited to participate in the study. Their DNA is studied for common genes. If hundreds of women are studied, each region of every chromosome can be examined, and it can be determined which genes are shared by the sisters who share the fibroid phenotype but are different in many other respects. This approach often produces novel genes that were not previously thought to be involved in the disease process.

Working in the laboratory of my colleague, Dr. Cynthia Morton, we are completing our collection of families for a genome-wide scan, called the Finding Genes for Fibroids study (www.fibroids.net). We hope within the next few years to identify genes that may be involved in fibroids.[28] Because our prior work suggests that African American women have different genes causing fibroids, an important part of the Finding Genes for Fibroids study is making sure that half of the women in our study are African American. We need to find these genes that make fibroids so common and so severe in black women.

CHAPTER 18

Pregnancy, Infertility, and Miscarriage

The most difficult question my patients ask me is, "Will my fibroid interfere with a pregnancy?" Since fibroids are so common, many women have absolutely normal pregnancies without even knowing they have fibroids. There are several different ways in which pregnancy may be affected by fibroids, however. Many women ask:

"Will the fibroid interfere with my getting pregnant?"
"Will the fibroid increase my risk of miscarriage?"
"Will the fibroid lead to other pregnancy complications?"
"If I want to treat the fibroid, will the treatment I choose create problems for a pregnancy?"

It is a good idea to ask all the questions and weigh the risks and benefits of intervening for fibroids.

Early Pregnancy Problems: Infertility and Early Miscarriage

It has been estimated that between 25 and 75 percent of all women have fibroids; clearly, then, many women have fibroids during a pregnancy and while they are trying for a pregnancy. Before ultrasound was widely used, many pregnant women, in fact, would not know that they had fibroids. However, with increasing use of ultrasound and improvements in ultrasound technology, many women are found to have a fibroid before pregnancy or in early pregnancy.

Since there is so much variability in fibroid behavior, if you have never tried for pregnancy and you have an asymptomatic fibroid, you can probably start trying for pregnancy without concern. (It is always a good idea to discuss your plans for pregnancy with your gynecologist because preconception counseling can help women have a healthy pregnancy.)

Fibroids generally grow during pregnancy, although some stay the same size and others shrink. Thus women whose fibroid is discovered during pregnancy may have had it for a while before it was found.

If you have trouble getting pregnant, however, or you have problems with miscarriage, the situation needs to be investigated. Generally we recommend that couples without risk factors for infertility seek evaluation for infertility if they have been trying for pregnancy for a year without success. Trying for a year is a good benchmark if your only experience of a fibroid is that one has been identified on an ultrasound or pelvic exam.

However, if you have factors that make you more likely to have infertility problems, most physicians recommend that couples seek a gynecologist's advice after 6 months of trying for pregnancy. The most common reason for an earlier evaluation is that the woman is 35 years old or older, but this advice also applies to other factors affecting fertility, such as a woman having irregular periods or a man having previous chemotherapy. If you have fibroid symptoms or if you have had fibroid treatment, then I would recommend seeking evaluation at 6 months.

Most gynecologists conduct a basic infertility evaluation for their patients, and some also offer fertility treatment. A urologist also can participate in the evaluation of men with infertility. However, within the discipline of obstetrics and gynecology there are gynecologists who have additional training and certification (subspecialists) in reproductive endocrinology and infertility (REI subspecialists). These REI subspecialists generally offer comprehensive infertility evaluation and services. The Internet provides additional information regarding the certification process (www.abog.org/women/women. html) or locating an REI subspecialist (www.socrei.org/).

A fibroid should never be implicated as the primary underlying problem when a woman has problems with infertility or miscarriage.

A thorough evaluation of the woman and her partner must be carried out first. The fibroid may not be a factor in the difficulty in conception or carrying the pregnancy, or there may be several different factors, including a fibroid, working together.

An early miscarriage (during the first 3 months of pregnancy) occurs very commonly. Most early miscarriages are due to genetic problems in the fetus (chromosomal, or karyotypic, abnormality). The events that must take place for an egg and sperm to develop into the fetus and its placenta are so complicated that often a chromosome or piece of chromosome is lost or added during the earliest development period, which leads to miscarriage. Some miscarriages occur so early that women assume they are not getting pregnant when, in fact, they may be losing the pregnancy before their missed period.[1] So even in women with fibroids, most early miscarriages are not due to the fibroids.

However, just as with heavy menstrual bleeding, assessing the position of the fibroid is critical for determining whether there is an increased risk of early pregnancy problems. There is reasonably good evidence that fibroids that distort the endometrium (submucosal fibroids) lead to increased risk of infertility and miscarriage.[2]

In 1984, a major study suggested that submucosal leiomyomas were related to infertility.[3] In this study, the pregnancy rate among women with at least 3 years of infertility and no other infertility factors who had a submucosal fibroid resected was more than 60 percent in the first year following resection. At the time hysteroscopic myomectomy was not yet available, so an abdominal myomectomy was done even for Type 0 and I fibroids. Thus, this high rate of success takes into account problems with adhesion formation (scar tissue) following abdominal surgery but reflects only a small number of patients and highly skilled surgeons.

Nonetheless, an abdominal myomectomy is a major surgical procedure, and many woman and doctors consider it as the last resort to optimize chances of pregnancy. Luckily, as hysteroscopic myomectomy was introduced, many women had an easier option; the impact of many Type 0 and I submucosal fibroids on pregnancy could be eliminated with fewer risks and a shorter recovery.

As in vitro fertilization (IVF) became more widely used for fertility treatment, a number of studies looked at women with leiomyomas and assessed the impact of fibroids on pregnancy outcome following this procedure. Most of the studies have, indeed, shown an adverse impact of myomas on fertility outcomes.[4,5] However, there is a clear bias in these studies. The general feeling is that prior to an expensive and invasive treatment option such as IVF, any strategy to maximize pregnancy rates should be employed. This is especially true because in most states insurance does not cover infertility treatment but does cover fibroid surgery. The fact that women, then, are allowed to proceed with an IVF cycle with a fibroid in place may suggest that the difficulty of removing this myoma is increased because of another problem or that the fibroid is a recurrent fibroid after conservative therapy.

We also cannot exclude the possibility that fibroids are not the true cause of pregnancy problems but instead just a marker of myometrial dysfunction. The reason this distinction is important is that if fibroids are the *result* of an underlying myometrial problem, removing them would not improve pregnancy outcome. Alternatively, if fibroids were the underlying *cause*, surgical removal may lead to better outcomes.

In addition, the earlier studies that suggested that distortion of the endometrial cavity led to poor pregnancy outcomes were substantiated. In IVF cycles, the chance of implantation was increased at least threefold in the presence of a normal endometrial cavity as opposed to an abnormal cavity.[4] An extension of this concept that myomas interfered with fertility, IVF, and other assisted reproductive technologies was published in 1998.[5] This study showed a hierarchy in which submucosal fibroids led to the lowest pregnancy rate, subserosal fibroids to the highest rate, and intramural fibroids an intermediate level, suggesting that the distance between the fibroid and the endometrial cavity somehow controlled the chance of pregnancy.

Late Pregnancy Problems: Second-Trimester Pregnancy Loss and Pregnancy Complications

Most miscarriages occur early in pregnancy. However, late miscarriages do (rarely) occur during the fourth and fifth month of pregnancy (second trimester). These miscarriages are often more difficult than early miscarriages both physically and emotionally. These late miscarriages are often related to uterine problems, including fibroids, and not to chromosome problems. Other uterine problems that can lead to second-trimester miscarriage include developmental problems in the mother such as a uterine septum or various forms of a double uterus. (The uterus is formed early during fetal life, when the two sides of the uterus fuse together. If there is a problem with this process, various forms of uterine duplication occur.)

Even if fibroids do not cause infertility or miscarriage, they may cause complications of pregnancy. The earliest large study of this issue, published in 1989, looked back at pregnancies in more than 6,000 women, of whom 1.4 percent had fibroids on pre-pregnancy ultrasounds.[6] At that time ultrasound imaging was not as precise as it currently is, and many fibroids would have been missed. The most important finding of this study, however, was that the risk of placental abruption occurred in approximately 60 percent of the pregnancies in which the fibroid was directly underneath the placenta. In a placental abruption, the placenta separates from the uterine wall before delivery. Unfortunately, half of these placental abruptions also produced fetal death. This compares with only 2.5 percent of patients having an abruption when the fibroid was in a different position in the uterus. This clearly pointed to a problem of abnormal placental function when the placenta was implanted over a large fibroid.

It is not clear why this occurs, but we can again consider the analogy of trying to grow a tree in shallow soil overlying a large rock. Also in this study, the risk of premature labor was increased in about 20 percent of these pregnancies, and about 15 percent of women had pain substantial enough to require narcotics. Both of these outcomes were more likely as the size of fibroid increased. Therefore, it appears that both the size of the fibroid and the location of the placenta are important in predicting the chance of pregnancy complications. This study also found an increased risk of cesarean section. There was no evidence that fetal growth was affected.

A second study looking at pregnancy complications due to fibroids has the advantage of being a population-based study rather than a review of hospital records.[7] More than 2,000 women were studied in this report, and adjustment was made for other factors that might coexist with fibroids. These findings were consistent with the ones from the earlier study. In the population-based study, the risk of bleeding during the first trimester was almost doubled, and the risk of placental abruption was increased almost by a factor of four. In addition, the possibility that the baby presented in breach presentation (feet or buttocks first rather than head first), which today largely requires a C-section delivery, was increased fourfold. The possibility of dysfunction during labor (where uterine contractions are not very effective) was doubled, and the risk of a C-section was increased by a factor of six.

Fibroid Treatments and Pregnancy

Even if there are increased risks of infertility, miscarriage, and pregnancy complications with fibroids, that does not mean that all fibroids should be surgically removed. The complications and side effects of the treatment may outweigh the benefits. For example, the problems with adhesion formation (scar tissue) following surgery may outweigh the benefit of removing the fibroid. In addition, removing the fibroid may not entirely correct the problem; the fibroid may be the result of a more basic problem in the normal muscle and not the true cause of pregnancy problems. Finally, the side effects of a less complicated procedure may be worth accepting, whereas those of a more involved procedure may not.

When faced with making a decision about whether to proceed with removal of a fibroid, women must consider the advantages and disadvantages of the surgical or interventional procedure. All surgical removals include the standard surgical risks, such as excessive bleeding, postoperative infection, risk of anesthesia, and risk of blood clots in the legs or lungs due to decreased ambulation after the surgery. These complications occur rarely because women with fibroids tend to be otherwise young and healthy. They are nonetheless factors to consider in the balance of risks and benefits.

The risk of postoperative surgical adhesions or scar tissue is clearly a major issue when fertility is the goal. Most studies have shown high rates of adhesion formation, but the degree of adhesions is often difficult to assess, since a second surgery must be done to visualize adhesions from a prior surgery. Some adhesions are thin and transparent like spider webs, and others are thick bands similar to shoelaces. At times the scarring can be so severe that it looks like the pelvis was once covered with glue so that all the structures are so stuck together that it's impossible to tell where one begins and the other ends.

The bowel can be stuck to the uterus and ovaries so that it is difficult to see where one tissue begins and the other ends, or the open end of the fallopian tube can be "glued shut." The type, amount, and location of adhesions determine their impact on fertility. Minimizing adhesion formation is an important goal, as we discussed in the chapter on surgical therapies (Chapter 10). However, the impact of adhesions on fertility has changed over time. Before options such as IVF were available, a woman whose fallopian tubes became blocked as a result of adhesions had no chance of pregnancy. Now, however, with these newer fertility techniques, pregnancy may still be possible if a woman has blocked fallopian tubes. Of course, most women would rather be able to become pregnant without medical interventions, so the risk of adhesions must be taken into account.

There are specific risks to specific fibroid procedures that go beyond general surgical risks. The first of these is the risk of uterine rupture, which appears to be elevated following laparoscopic myomectomy or myolysis (uterine rupture is discussed in Chapter 9). Long-term studies of women undergoing laparoscopic myomectomy and seeking fertility would help us better understand this risk of uterine rupture. Available evidence suggests that *fertility rates* (the ability to become pregnant) after laparoscopic myomectomy are good, however. A woman should discuss these important issues with her doctor before proceeding with a laparoscopic myomectomy when she desires fertility.

Hysteroscopic myomectomy does not appear to be associated with a similar risk of uterine rupture. In addition, numerous studies suggest that there is no impairment of fertility following hysteroscopic myomectomy. Although intrauterine adhesions can sometimes occur following hysteroscopic surgery, this appears to be a rare event, and the benefits of removing the fibroid and normalizing the endometrial cavity appear to outweigh this risk.

The latest interventional treatment that appears to have a specific impact on women desiring fertility is uterine artery embolization (UAE). Although UAE provides successful treatment for some women, it does have an impact on fertility. The earliest case series reported that between 5 and 8 percent of women had enough ovarian dysfunction following the procedure to stop having periods. In the largest Canadian study, where more than 500 women were followed, it appears that this outcome is strongly age-related. In women who are under 40 years of age, there is less than a 4 percent chance of having ovarian failure.[8] However, in women over 50, this risk rises to 40 percent.

What causes this ovarian damage? It was originally thought to be due purely to the placement of the embolic pellets in the ovarian blood vessels rather than in the uterine blood vessels, where they are meant to be placed. Although this can happen, knowledge of the anatomy of the pelvis suggests that it is not necessarily the reason that the ovaries are damaged by UAE. If the uterine arteries are occluded (blocked), the uterus would likely "recruit" the secondary blood supply through the ovarian blood vessels. This could leave the ovary vulnerable to changes caused by decreased blood supply and could impair fertility by depriving some ovarian follicles of their blood supply.

There is evidence that the ovarian failure is sometimes transient and that even women who have elevated gonadotropins (follicle-stimulating hormone, or FSH, and luteinizing hormone, or LH) consistent with menopause can resume cycling. The question for women seeking fertility is whether there might be significant destruction of eggs even if they continue having normal cycles. This situation is termed *decreased ovarian reserve* and can result in difficulty getting pregnant. (Decreased ovarian reserve is the most common reason older women, even without UAE, have difficulty getting pregnant.)

In addition, there is controversy about whether women who have had UAE are more likely to have poor pregnancy outcomes. A large study of women undergoing UAE has suggested that there may be an increased risk of placental problems in pregnancies following UAE.[9] We know that these placental problems are more common in women who have had prior pregnancies and especially prior C-sections. Because the women in this report had not had prior C-sections, it may be that, like C-section, UAE affects the uterine wall in a way that makes it harder for the placenta to find the right place to implant. More studies are needed, but until then we say that UAE is not often the first choice for the woman who wants to have children. When other risks and benefits are taken into account, however, UAE may be a good option. For example, if a woman has had complications following a prior myomectomy, or if she has medical issues that would increase her risk of complications from surgery, UAE may be the appropriate fertility-preserving option.

Additional studies of fibroids in pregnancy are clearly necessary. Until we have more information, many women will be making their decision with incomplete information. Your preferences and the experience of your physician also weigh into the decision.

I do feel strongly that as new therapies are developed they should first be tested in women who do not desire future fertility. This is the approach we took in designing the studies of magnetic resonance imaging (MRI)–guided focused ultrasound surgery (MRgFUS). Although the benefits of new minimally invasive therapies are often easily seen, the risks may not be apparent until later. Additionally some new therapies present significant safety problems that may lead to hysterectomy. I believe it is a better strategy to test innovative therapies on women who are not interested in childbearing and, once safety and efficacy have been established, to extend the therapies to women desiring fertility.

CHAPTER 19

Adenomyosis and Endometrial Polyps

Adenomyosis

Adenomyosis, like fibroids, is a benign disease of the uterus. Some women have adenomyosis and fibroids, and sometimes adenomyosis is mistaken for fibroids. When adenomyosis results in a large mass in the uterine wall (called an *adenomyoma*), the condition can seem to be very similar to fibroids. However, under the microscope, the tissue appears very different.

Fibroids, as we know, are composed of smooth muscle, and there is a distinct dividing line, called a *pseudocapsule*, between the fibroid and the surrounding normal myometrium. Adenomyosis, in constrast, is composed of tissue that looks like the lining of the uterus (fig. 19.1). The glands and the stroma (the supporting tissue) intertwine with the myometrial cells and make it difficult to separate the adenomyosis from the uterus. In this way the condition is similar to endometriosis, and, in fact, an older term for adenomyosis was *endometriosis interna* (or endometriosis inside the muscle). The adenomyosis tissue leads to growth (hypertrophy) of the normal myometrium surrounding "nests" of endometrial tissue.

Some women do not have a large collection of adenomyosis in their uterine wall but instead have microscopic areas that resemble the uterine lining scattered throughout the uterine wall. This condi-

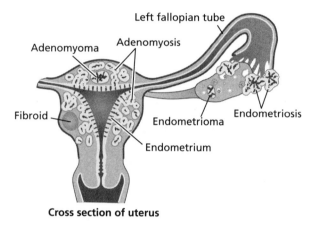

Cross section of uterus

Surfaces, viewed from the front

Figure 19.1. Adenomyosis is a condition in which tissue that looks like endometrium is found inside the muscle layer of the uterus. It can form fibroid-like nodules called adenomyomas. Adenomyomas are more deeply infiltrating into the myometrium than fibroids. Because they don't have a clear layer surrounding them from the myometrium, adenomyomas are more difficult to remove surgically than fibroids. Adenomyosis can also be diffuse, and in that case, small areas of microscopic adenomyosis are scattered throughout the myometrium. Endometriosis is another disease where tissue that appears to be like endometrium is in the wrong place. Endometriosis occurs when this tissue is found on the pelvic surfaces or the ovaries. Endometriosis deep inside the ovary is termed an endometrioma and can sometimes be invisible from the surface of the ovary. Sometimes endometriosis can lead to the formation of adhesions or scar tissue that can cause effects even after the endometriosis is successfully treated. Previously adenomyosis was called *endometriosis interna* because of this similarity, but we now believe adenomyosis and endometriosis are distinctly different diseases.

tion is called *diffuse adenomyosis,* and it is currently even more difficult to treat surgically than adenomyomas.

Women with adenomyosis and women with uterine fibroids both tend to have periods that are long or heavy or both (menorrhagia). Both of these conditions are also most likely found in women in their forties and fifties who are premenopausal.

How, then, can we tell whether a woman has adenomyosis instead of uterine fibroids?[1,2] There are some clues.

The first is that, in classic cases, the uterus with adenomyosis is not irregular on the outside, as is the case with subserosal fibroids, but is enlarged and softened, more like a pregnant uterus. The terms *boggy* and *globular* (like a globe) are more often used to describe the uterus with adenomyosis than a uterus with fibroids. Women with adenomyosis are also more likely to have painful periods (dysmenorrhea). There is also some evidence that painful periods are more likely when the adenomyosis goes deep into the uterine wall.

Studies of women with adenomyosis also suggest that women who have had multiple pregnancies are more likely to have adenomyosis. In contrast, having multiple pregnancies appears to protect women from developing fibroids. Because until recently the diagnosis of adenomyosis was made only after hysterectomy, this association of adenomyosis with an increasing number of pregnancies may be spurious. It may be that because women who have had pregnancies are more willing to undergo a hysterectomy, they may be the only ones who will be diagnosed with surgically proven adenomyosis.

There are similarities between the molecules important to fibroids and the molecules important to adenomyosis. Factors that promote blood vessel growth or scar tissue formation, as well as prolactin (another hormone produced by the pituitary), appear to be important in both diseases.[3]

Again, as with fibroids, we do not know how adenomyosis forms. The most commonly held theory is that the uterine lining "invades" the normal myometrium and then produces the surrounding excess growth of the myometrium (hypertrophy). However, this is just a theory. It may be, instead, either that the adenomyosis formed during fetal development, prior to birth, or that normal cell types change (metaplasia) to endometrium-like cells as a result of local factors. Studies are beginning to suggest that one of these other theories may be more likely to explain adenomyosis than the direct invasion pathway.[3,4]

As mentioned above, adenomyosis is primarily diagnosed following surgery, when the uterine tissue can be examined under a microscope. Both ultrasound and magnetic resonance imaging (MRI) can be useful, although MRI appears to be much more likely to correctly diagnose adenomyosis than ultrasound (plate 7).[5,6] Knowing whether you have adenomyosis before you decide to have certain procedures, such as abdominal myomectomy and uterine artery embolization (UAE), may be important. Minimally invasive treatments are generally less effective for adenomyosis than they are for fibroids.

Traditionally, the treatment for adenomyosis has been hysterectomy. A skilled surgeon, however, can resect (remove) specific areas of adenomyosis in the uterine wall; this type of procedure is similar to a myomectomy. Generally it is a temporary measure, however, since adenomyosis is inevitably left behind.

Therapy with a gonadotropin-releasing hormone (GnRH) agonist will also provide short-term relief of symptoms but is not likely to give long-term relief. This therapy has been used on a short-term basis for some women, some of whom have then become pregnant after the GnRh agonist therapy ended. Finally, a recent report suggests that a medicated intrauterine device (IUD) containing the medication danazol (a synthetic androgen) has been useful in the treatment of symptoms.[7] This device is not currently available commercially, however.

UAE has been used to treat adenomyosis but it is generally less successful than when it is used for the treatment of fibroids. Hysterectomy is still the gold standard treatment option for adenomyosis, but UAE may sometimes be the right treatment.

Many important questions need to be answered about adenomyosis. Many women have both fibroids and adenomyosis, which makes it even more difficult to determine which symptoms are caused by each disease. Since these diseases share some of the same molecular changes, are they different manifestations of the same process? Unfortunately, we have few answers at this time.

Endometrial Polyps

Endometrial polyps are another benign growth of the uterus that can cause problems with menstrual bleeding. Unlike fibroids and adenomyosis, however, endometrial polyps begin in the endometrium (the uterine lining) and stay within the endometrial layer (fig. 19.2).

Endometrial polyps may be fingerlike projections, similar to polyps in the intestine, or they may be more rounded, in which case they may be hard to distinguish from fibroids. Generally, polyps and fibroids lead to different symptoms. Polyps usually cause irregular bleeding (metorrhagia) or irregular bleeding that is also heavy at times (menometorrhagia), but they do not cause the long, heavy bleeding (menorrhagia) associated with fibroids or adenomyosis.[3] They also do not usually cause pain. It is currently controversial whether they play a role in infertility.[8]

Although most polyps are found in postmenopausal women, between 10 and 25 percent of premenopausal women who are undergoing evaluation or treatment for abnormal bleeding are found

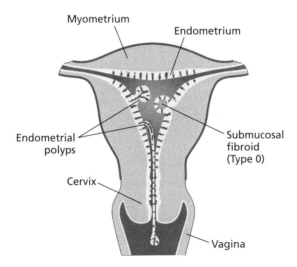

Figure 19.2. A polyp arises out of the endometrial layer of the uterus, whereas a fibroid arises from the muscle layer. It is therefore possible to remove a polyp by scraping the inside of the uterus during a D&C (dilation and curettage) or by grasping it with a pair of tongs (polyp forceps). However, it is difficult to know for sure whether all polyps have been removed without looking inside the uterus directly with a hysteroscope or indirectly with a sonohysterogram. The polyp pictured in the left of the image can be difficult to distinguish from the submucosal fibroid on the right by sonohysterogram. Polyps can also sometimes prolapse (fall through) through the cervix and be visible when looking at the cervix.

to have polyps.[9,10] There is also evidence that women without symptoms may have polyps, but these polyps tend to be smaller and more likely to regress (disappear without treatment) than polyps in women with symptoms.[11,12]

Because they are confined to the endometrial layer, polyps are easier to remove than submucous fibroids of the same size. I think of the difference between them as the difference between the polyp, which is located in the layer that is normally "peeled off" during menstruation, and the fibroid, which is firmly "bolted" to the myometrial wall. Although polyps may be removed by dilation and curettage (D&C), a scraping of the inside of the uterus, they can be more difficult to remove in this way than many gynecologists believe. Until gynecologists had the ability to look inside the uterus with a hysteroscope after completing a D&C, they didn't realize what they had missed. Paradoxically, gynecologists sometimes also miss polyps because they are so big. During a hysteroscopy a large polyp can be so big that it looks like the wall of the uterus.

Many physicians combine a D&C with the use of a clamp called a polyp forcep to reach blindly into the uterus to grab the polyps, but this is not as effective a treatment as one that allows the physician to see the inside of the uterus. Studies suggest that utilizing hysteroscopy gives better results than the blind D&C for diagnosing structural lesions like polyps that are causing bleeding.[13,14]

Although it is often assumed that polyps become a major problem with women after menopause, studies suggest that premenopausal women are as likely to have polyps as postmenopausal women. Postmenopausal women who develop abnormal uterine bleeding are more likely to seek medical care quickly because of concern about cancer of the endometrium, and therefore they are more likely to be diagnosed with polyps, which are discovered as part of the investigation into the cause of the bleeding.

Polyps can be a particular problem for women undergoing tamoxifen treatment for breast cancer because their polyps tend to become quite large. If the ongoing studies of tamoxifen for breast cancer prevention show this is a good treatment for more and younger women, then more and younger women may develop large polyps.

CHAPTER 20

Uterine Cancers

There are two basic types of uterine cancers. The first and much more common type is cancer of the uterine lining, or endometrial cancer, a type of adenocarcinoma. Endometrial cancers typically cause abnormal uterine bleeding. This is the primary reason that doctors are quick to perform an endometrial biopsy to exclude the possibility of endometrial cancer when women have bleeding between periods or postmenopausal bleeding. The risk of endometrial cancer increases with increasing age and for women after menopause.[1,2] There are other risk factors for endometrial cancer, as well. Risk of endometrial cancer is increased in women who are obese and do not ovulate regularly, women who have high blood pressure or diabetes, and women who have never had a child.[1,2] Each of these conditions is thought to result in an excess of estrogen, which causes the endometrial lining to grow. This is why estrogen alone is seldom given to a woman with a uterus; it is usually combined with progesterone or a progestin to limit the growth of the lining. Additionally, physicians are much more likely to do a biopsy in women who have any of these risk factors than in women who have none but who have some irregular bleeding.

The rarer type of cancer is a cancer of the muscle, or a sarcoma. There are many different kinds of sarcomas, such as carcinosarcoma, leiomyosarcoma and endometrial stromal sarcoma. Each different type of sarcoma has a distinct tissue pattern when viewed under the microscope; by examining this pattern we both determine the kind of sarcoma and get a sense of how it will behave. In the future, as with other cancers, we will not depend on the microscopic pattern but will instead look for specific molecular markers (molecules made by the tumors that identify them and tell us how aggressively they will behave and how to best treat them). Sarcomas are the kind of cancer that is often confused with fibroids, since both diseases can be felt as a nodule in the wall of the uterus.

To be 100 percent certain that a woman has a fibroid and not a sarcoma, the tumor must be removed and examined under a microscope. This is generally not a wise way to proceed, however. A woman who is suspected to have fibroids has a risk of having a uterine sarcoma that is at most 1 in 10,000, but the risk of a significant complication during surgery is 1 in 1,000. Therefore, for most women, the risk of having an iatrogenic complication (one caused by the procedure) outweighs the chance of finding a cancer. For this reason the American College of Obstetricians and Gynecologists recommends that concern about cancer should not be the only reason to proceed with a hysterectomy for a woman with uterine fibroids.[3] Rarely cancers will be missed with this strategy, but many women will be spared significant complications from surgery.

Although it is possible to stick a needle into many fibroids and obtain a small piece of tissue to view under a microscope, this, too, is generally not a wise way to proceed for most women.[4] Distinguishing between a sarcoma and a fibroid involves looking at many different criteria in a number of different areas of the tumor, including

- the number of dividing cells over many different areas of the tumor (mitoses per high power field of magnification);
- the appearance of the cells (atypia); and
- the extent and the pattern of dead cells (necrosis).

Distinguishing between a sarcoma and a fibroid is so difficult that there are tumors that don't fit into either category and that are classified as leiomyomas of uncertain malignant potential (UMP), as we discuss in Chapter 21. Because pathologists need to look at many different areas to be certain that the tumor is a sarcoma, a frozen section diagnosis (one obtained by quickly freezing tissue and examining it while the surgery is going on) is not as reliable as with other tumors, so doctors are not certain of the diagnosis until the full report is ready several days later. It can be a frustrating wait for a woman and her family, but it is important to have the correct information.

Most medical textbooks teach that rapid growth of a uterine mass should make the physician suspect that it is a sarcoma rather than a fibroid. Not only is there no agreement on what amount of growth is too much, but there is no evidence that rapid growth is associated with sarcomas.[5-7] Many fibroids can grow rapidly, and unnecessary surgeries are sometimes performed because of concern regarding growth.

For a woman who has specific factors that increase the risk of sarcoma, surgery may be justified. The risk of sarcomas increases with increasing age, regardless of menopause status. Thus an 80-year-old woman with a uterine mass may be more likely to have a sarcoma than a 65-year-old woman with a uterine mass, even though both women are in menopause. Therefore, a woman who develops a new uterine mass after menopause, particularly after some time in the postmenopausal period, is more likely to make the physician suspect a diagnosis of a sarcoma than a younger woman, who is more likely to have fibroids.

Some women who may have had silent or asymptomatic fibroids have their first ultrasound near the time of menopause and may mistakenly be thought to have a new, suspicious uterine mass. Waiting and watching is a reasonable decision in this case, rather than deciding to have immediate surgery. If the mass stays the same size or shrinks over time, it is most likely a fibroid. If it grows, further diagnostic imaging or treatment may be the best course.

Black women appear to be more likely to have sarcomas than white women, just as they are more likely to have fibroids.[8] Besides race, other risk factors for uterine sarcomas include prior radiation therapy of the pelvis (in which the uterus would have been exposed to radiation) and use of tamoxifen.[9] As discussed previously, women who have the rare genetic syndrome hereditary leiomyomatosis and renal cell carcinoma (HLRCC) appear to be at risk for a sarcoma, which may develop at an early age. A physician will be more likely to suspect a sarcoma if he or she feels a uterine mass on pelvic exam in a 62-year-old black woman who has previously been treated with tamoxifen for breast cancer than in a 35-year-old woman without these additional risk factors. This increased suspicion may lead to more or different diagnostic testing (such as ordering magnetic resonance imaging, or MRI, rather than an ultrasound as the first test) or a lower threshold for considering surgical treatment.

There are a few tests that may increase your physician's suspicion that you have cancer rather than a fibroid. In a series of women with sarcomas treated at the same institution, the cancer diagnosis of about a third of them had been made before surgery with an endometrial biopsy.[5] Although a normal biopsy does not eliminate the possibility of cancer, since it is a safe and easy test to perform, for most women it makes sense to have a biopsy before surgery for a presumed sarcoma.

MRI can also be useful in differentiating a sarcoma from a benign uterine leiomyoma.[10,11] Again, a normal MRI does not exclude the possibility of cancer, but particular patterns will alert your physician to an increased possibility of a cancer. Finally, scientists are looking at serum markers (proteins in the blood that indicate the disease, in this case a sarcoma, is present) to help distinguish fibroids from sarcomas. Currently these are done only as research studies, but they may be useful in the future.

Some reports suggest that sarcomas are less likely than fibroids to respond to conservative therapies such as gonadotropin-releasing hormone (GnRH) agonist and uterine artery embolization.[12-14] Therefore, if you don't respond to one of these minimally invasive therapies, you have to think carefully about whether there are benefits to having a hysterectomy for definitive treatment and diagnosis. All these tests provide clues rather than absolute proof of the presence or absence of a sarcoma. Even a mass that grows rapidly in a postmenopausal woman may turn out to be a fibroid.[16] Alternatively, a sarcoma can be present in a young woman with no risk factors.

If you are having surgery for a suspected sarcoma, most doctors recommend that the ovaries should be removed as well, because some sarcomas respond to the steroid hormones estrogen and progesterone, produced by the ovaries. Your surgical plan should take this factor into consideration.

Finally, in the past, it was argued that fibroids should be removed when they reach a specified size so that an ovarian cancer would not be missed.[15] This is the same reason that an ultrasound examination should be done if fibroids are suspected on the basis of a pelvic exam: the lumpy, irregular feel of a fibroid uterus can be confused with a mass in the ovaries. The clarity of ultrasound imaging has increased substantially over the past two decades, however, so it should not be necessary to have surgery to eliminate the possibility of an ovarian mass.

The more common problem is that the ovaries may not be seen on an ultrasound in the presence of large fibroids. Fibroids and ovaries look very different on ultrasound, but the fibroids may be pushing the ovaries into an atypical position so that they are hard to see. Because ovarian cancers generally cause the ovaries to be larger than normal ovaries, not seeing the ovaries is usually a reassuring sign, but, again, there is never a guarantee.

In the twenty-first century surgeons seldom remove organs to prevent them from becoming cancerous. We have even moved away from routinely taking out the appendix when a person is undergoing unrelated abdominal surgery, unless there is a specific reason to do so. The exception to this rule is when a specific problem such as a genetic mutation (such as BRCA1 or BRCA2) substantially increases the risk of disease (breast and ovarian cancer). Even in this case, some women choose to have their ovaries (prophylactic oophorectomy) and/or breasts (prophylactic mastectomy) removed, and other women do not. Women make their choices based on many factors, including their experience with family members with these cancers, concerns about the disfigurement of surgery, and their work and family situations. Because you will have to accept the consequences of your decision, you need to participate in the decision-making process.

Having HLRCC syndrome is the only analogous situation we have with fibroids. Women who have the *fumarate hydratase* (*FH*) mutation causing this syndrome appear to have an increased risk of forming a sarcoma. Unfortunately, because we have only recently recognized this syndrome, we have little information to offer women as a guide in their decision-making process. We don't know whether the risk of cancer is increased 10 percent or 50 percent or 90 percent. Even in this case, each woman needs to make her own decisions. However, for the woman who has symptoms from her fibroids and who has decided on treatment, knowing this additional information about her genetic makeup may help tip the balance toward hysterectomy. The weighing of risks and benefits here is similar to that for the woman with symptomatic fibroids and problems with human papilloma virus (HPV) and abnormal Pap smears. For her situation, a hysterectomy solves two problems, whereas a myomectomy only solves one.

No one should be scared into having a hysterectomy. If your doctor says you need a hysterectomy because the fibroids "could be cancerous," review the information you have. Do you have risk factors? Is anything suspicious in the imaging? Does the MRI report state "highly suspicious for a sarcoma" or only "cannot exclude a sarcoma"? Does your doctor or does your hospital see a high volume of women with similar situations? If you have any questions, seeking a second opinion can be a good idea. Most large hospitals can arrange an appointment with a specialist right away so that a woman suspected of having cancer doesn't have a long wait for an appointment.

CHAPTER 21

Fibroid-like Conditions

Even if you assume that all fibroids behave like one disease (which, as we have seen, is unlikely to be true), there are several fibroid-like conditions that fall into a clearly different category.[1] Some of the features of these diseases appear to be fibroid-like, and some are more like cancerous tumors. Needless to say, because these diseases are rare, we know even less about them than we do about more typical fibroids. Understanding this in-between group, however, may help us better understand both fibroids and cancers as well as these fibroid-like conditions. There are several different diseases based on descriptive characteristics; however, it will be important to study them scientifically. They may truly be different diseases; some may be subsets of the same disease.

Intravenous Leiomyomatosis

Intravenous leiomyomatosis (IVL), like fibroids, affects only women. IVL is found in both premenopausal and postmenopausal women.

With IVL, the fibroids extend out from the uterus in a "wormlike" (vermiform) fashion through the blood vessels. At its greatest extent IVL can reach all the way from the uterus through the vascular system to the heart. This extension from the uterus to the heart can lead to a number of problems, such as a heart murmur, shortness of breath (dyspnea), heart palpitations, blood clots of the major blood vessels (thrombosis), fainting (syncope), leg swelling, or evidence of right-sided heart failure.

Sometimes IVL is diagnosed when women who have previously had a hysterectomy are found to have tissue extending from the pelvis to the heart. This disease is also sometimes first recognized when women are seen by a cardiac surgeon for removal of a mass in the heart (intracardiac mass).[2] The fact that women don't need to have a uterus at the time that IVL develops suggests that something more complicated is occurring than simply having the "fibroid-like" tissue move from the uterus into the blood vessels. Perhaps the abnormal cells that will form IVF can remain quiescent (quiet or silent) in the blood vessels and be triggered to grow at a later date. Alternatively, whatever stimulates these leiomyoma-like lesions to form in the uterus may stimulate independent formation of IVL in the blood vessels. Further research is necessary to understand this apparent paradox.

The disease may be recognized during what initially seems like a routine hysterectomy, when fibroid-like tissue starting in the uterus extends outward into the blood vessels supplying the uterus. IVL sometimes is recognized only at the time of pathology evaluation.[3] In fact, in my practice, a woman whose procedure I believed at the time of surgery to be just an extremely difficult myomectomy with much distortion due to scar tissue from a prior uterine surgery was found to have IVL based on chromosome analysis.

One study has described a tumor measuring 40 cm (18 inches) going from the uterine blood vessels through the inferior vena cava (which brings blood back from the lower body into the heart) all the way to the heart.[4] Although in many cases two surgeries are performed to take care of the disease in the pelvis and the disease in the chest, in some cases gynecologists and cardiovascular surgeons have worked together to remove all the IVL at the same time. With one surgical procedure, the gynecologists can remove the uterus, while the cardiac surgeons remove the heart and blood vessel disease through a separate chest incision using a heart bypass machine.[4]

IVL, like ordinary fibroids, appears to be a hormonally responsive disease and has been shown to regress with therapy using a gonadotropin-releasing hormone (GnRH) agonist.[5,6] IVL doesn't seem to disappear in these instances, merely to shrink so that surgical treatment is more feasible or disease remaining after surgery can be kept at a minimal level. Generally the vascular disease is removed surgically to prevent some of the more serious complications such as major blood clots.

No one is sure how IVL develops. One theory speculates that the disease arises from the extension and invasion of uterine leiomyomas into the smooth muscle cells of the blood vessels; another theory says that the smooth muscle cells of the vessels give rise to leiomyomas. Since the disease never appears in men, the first theory appears to be more likely. However, the second theory would better explain IVL in women following hysterectomy (discussed earlier).

A particular rearrangement of chromosomes 12 and 14 appears to be associated with IVL.[7] Intravenous leiomyomatosis thus appears to be related to the subgroup of ordinary fibroids that have the chromosome translocations involving chromosomes 12 and 14. Further molecular changes may lead to the more aggressive behavior of IVL. This genetic information also favors the theory that the disease starts with leiomyomas that then become more aggressive through an unknown mechanism.

Leiomyomatosis Peritonealis Disseminata

In leiomyomatosis peritonealis disseminata (LPD), multiple myoma-like nodules are present throughout the abdominal and pelvic cavity. Early reports primarily noted that LPD occurred in women who were pregnant or who were taking oral contraceptive pills. Although the average age of women in one series was 37, the condition has been described in women from 22 to 69 years of age. The diameter of lesions can range from 0.1 to 10 cm.[8]

At the time of surgery, the number of lesions seen in LPD and the distortion they cause in pelvic structure can make it seem like a cancerous process is occurring. Frozen section pathology at the time of surgery is sometimes helpful in sorting out the two processes. (LPD in very rare instances is found with malignancy.)[8]

Symptoms appear to wax and wane with LPD, and therefore regression of disease does occur—but recurrence at a later date is common. This makes it very difficult to assess treatments.

The LPD lesions appear to have receptors for estrogen and progesterone as well as luteinizing hormone (LH).[9,10] This may explain why women tend to develop LPD in pregnancy and while taking birth control pills, two states in which the body has high levels of estrogen and progesterone. A case report suggested that treatment with progestins was effective.[11] Even following hysterectomy and removal of both ovaries, recurrences of LPD have been reported in women taking estrogen and progestin hormone replacement therapy.[12]

Biologically, the lesions of LPD appear to be clonal tumors and to have some similarity to leiomyomas.[13] The guinea pig model of fibroids with multiple nodules throughout the abdomen may in fact be more similar to LPD than to ordinary fibroids (see Chapter 3).[14]

Lymphangioleiomyomatosis

Lymphangioleiomyomatosis (LAM) is the most serious fibroid-like disease. In LAM fibroid-like lesions are found in the lungs and can lead to significant destruction of lung tissue. This lung disease can be fatal. In LAM, the original tumor is not a fibroid but a similar benign tumor in the kidney, a renal angiomyolipoma.[15] The true inciting event is likely to be a mutation in the *tuberous sclerosis complex 2* (*TSC2*) gene.[16,17] This gene codes for the protein tubulin, which is a major component of cell structure and also appears to act as a tumor suppressor.

Mutations in the *TSC2* gene as well as a related gene, *TSC1*, cause tuberous sclerosis (TS), a disease that has noticeable overlap with LAM. In TS, many types of benign tumors may appear throughout the body. TS affects both sexes. The lung disease that people with TS develop appears to be the same process that takes place in women with LAM.

Although LAM appears to originate from a benign kidney tumor, it is entirely a disease of women. Most women who develop LAM are premenopausal (with an average age of 33 in one series), but LAM can be diagnosed after menopause, though this is rare.[18] There also appears to be a separate link between fibroids and LAM in that women with LAM were found to be more likely than other women to have a relative with uterine fibroids.[19]

Lung symptoms are the most common initial clues to LAM. Shortness of breath (dyspnea) is often an early symptom; coughing up blood (hemoptysis) is another symptom.[18,20,21] The disease leads to the formation of lung cysts and lung collapse, in which the space the lung occupied fills with air (pneumothorax) or fluid (chylothorax). The lung disease appears to be an interstitial pattern more like emphysema, in which the lymphatic spaces (located between the air spaces in the lung) are altered. The lymphatic system takes excess fluid that is located between cells and tissues and collects it into channels similar to blood vessels and eventually deposits the fluid directly into the bloodstream. The lymphatics and the blood vessels travel together in the lung between air spaces just as the pipes for plumbing run between walls and floors in a house; the space where they are located is termed the *interstitial space.*

Many methods of manipulating steroid hormones, including medications and oophorectomy (removing the ovaries), have been reported to stabilize or (rarely) improve LAM symptoms.[18,22–24] However, no treatment has been compared with a placebo treatment, and there are also reports of most therapies showing no effect. In one large series, the only drug that showed improvement in lung status was the progestin medroxyprogesterone acetate.[18,24]

Lung transplantation has been used as the last resort for the most severe LAM disease. However, LAM cells can cause new LAM lesions in the transplanted lung.[25,26]

LAM cells have both the alpha and beta versions of the estrogen receptor and androgen receptors, and estrogenic compounds like estrogen and tamoxifen have been shown to stimulate LAM cells in laboratory studies.[15] These receptors may in part explain why LAM is a hormonally responsive disease. There also appear to be abnormalities in the enzymes that degrade extracellular matrix (ECM) in LAM that leads to cysts forming in the lungs.[27] Just as with fibroids, control of the ECM may provide a future approach to treatment.

Benign Metastasizing Leiomyoma

Benign metastasizing leiomyoma (BML) is characterized by typical leiomyomas in the uterus and what appear to be fibroid-like lesions in a distant location, most often the lung.[28] BML behaves in a relatively benign fashion compared with the deterioration of lung function seen in LAM. In BML the fibroid-like lesions are present in the lung, but the distortion of the interstitial spaces, which leads to so many of the pulmonary problems in women with LAM, is not. There is some evidence that removing the ovaries can cure BML, whereas oophorectomy merely slows the progression of LAM.[22]

Leiomyomas of Uncertain Malignant Potential

Leiomyomas of uncertain malignant potential (UMP) is the easiest fibroid-like disease to understand because there are no associated findings elsewhere in the body. This diagnosis is based purely on the analysis of the fibroid tissue under the microscope. The tissue has some of the markers we associate with sarcomas, but not enough to meet the formal definition.[29,30]

Thus, physicians have to base their medical decisions and care on the nature of the findings (having one small area of concern is less worrisome than if there are multiple abnormal areas throughout the tumor) and the woman's clinical situation (recommending surgery to remove the ovaries is easier in a 52-year-old woman than in a 35-year-old woman who had her fibroids removed before trying for pregnancy).

In the future it is likely that specific molecular markers or gene chips (as discussed in Chapter 3) will be used to define the risk of future problems and that UMP will disappear as a category of disease. We will likely also be able to identify these particular fibroid variants when we understand genetics better.

For women with these unusual fibroid variants, finding expert medical advice can be difficult. A nonprofit foundation, the LAM Foundation, provides information for women with LAM via the Internet (www.thelamfoundation.org). Physicians who serve on the scientific advisory boards of organizations such as the LAM Foundation likely have a special interest in caring for patients with this disease or are knowledgeable about where to seek expert care.

For women with these other diseases, there are no similar foundations. One of my goals over the next decade is to provide better care for such women. Most gynecologists will see at most a handful of women with these fibroid-variant diseases over their career. Thus, although it is always easier to see a physician who is located close to your home, a disease like this often creates a situation in which traveling a distance may be helpful and worthwhile.

Contacting people who do research on these conditions may help you find a knowledgeable physician. Another option for finding care would be to call the nearest major hospital or medical school and ask for advice. Having a center where physicians specialize in these rare diseases would also help us find new treatment options. It is hard to learn what works when you see only one or two women with the disease over the course of your career.

CHAPTER 22

Alternative and Complementary Therapies

What are alternative and complementary therapies? The National Institutes of Health (NIH) defines them as "a group of diverse medical and health care systems, practices, and products that are not presently considered to be part of conventional medicine" (http://nccam.nih.gov). A significant movement is under way to test these therapies (sometimes called unproven therapies) in the same way that new drugs and new devices are tested. This is why the National Center for Complementary and Alternative Medicine (NCCAM) was created as a part of the NIH. Just because we don't understand why something works does not mean that it can't be safe and effective. How and why aspirin works was discovered more than a hundred years after the drug was first marketed, and the bark of the willow tree from which aspirin was first derived was used therapeutically for many hundreds of years before anyone knew about prostaglandin synthesis.

The Internet provides a marketplace for the sale of many alternative and complementary therapies for uterine fibroids. However, there are few, if any, studies testing these purported treatments. (One could argue that this is a common situation for fibroid therapies, but conventional fibroid therapies have been used widely by many practitioners who have reported their results in peer-reviewed publications.) The following are some warning signs regarding products that may not have been widely tested:

- Classification of the product as a dietary supplement. The U.S. Food and Drug Administration (FDA) does not require supplements to be proven effective, only to be proven safe. In fact, the FDA does not require manufacturers of supplements to contact the FDA before beginning sales. Therefore, these products are not likely to have undergone the rigorous testing you expect and need before taking a powerful treatment (www.cfsan.fda.gov/~dms/supplmnt.html).

- Reporting testimonials rather than data. A testimonial is one patient's report of how effective the treatment is. Since disease may get better on its own and individuals may want to believe that their chosen therapy is effective, even many individuals speaking about a product's effectiveness does not prove that the product is effective.

- Claims such as "natural, safe, and has no side effects" and "dissolves fibroids" sound too good to be true. Everything has side effects, and we are always weighing side effects against benefits. As the old saying goes, if it sounds too good to be true, it probably is.

- Detailed explanation of how the treatment might work but no references to evidence of how it works in women with fibroids. Coming up with a way a compound works is called "generating a hypothesis" and is the first step in the scientific method. However, testing the compound in many ways is required before concluding that an agent is effective.

Steps are generally taken to assess the effectiveness of more conventional therapies, and these can be used for testing alternative and complementary therapies, as well. First you need a valid endpoint. Some women may feel that their uterus is smaller after therapy, but if an ultrasound demonstrates that it has grown, most people would believe the ultrasound. Thus an imaging test like an ultrasound is generally believed to be a more valid endpoint than a self-report. Likewise for bleeding: measuring menstrual blood loss is believed to be a more valid endpoint than a woman reporting that her periods are lighter. It is difficult to collect all the pads and tampons used during a period and extract the blood from the cotton and other binding materials in order to measure blood loss. This procedure is done with some research studies, but generally researchers have moved to pictorial diaries or validated questionnaires. Pictorial diaries have pictures of pads and tampons, and by matching the staining on your sanitary product to the ones pictured, blood loss is estimated. Validated questionnaires ask questions, and (from previous work) we can document that the questionnaire is providing a good measure of the amount of bleeding.

A standard part of testing any new treatment involves using a control or comparison group. Without a control group to eliminate the possibility of a placebo effect or spontaneous worsening or improvement in disease, effectiveness is difficult to demonstrate. For fibroids the control is relatively straightforward, since researchers can look at a number of treatments and assess a variety of endpoints. Commonly assessed endpoints include the size of fibroids (by ultrasound or other types of imaging), the amount of bleeding (with questionnaires, diaries, or blood counts), and quality of life (by questionnaires such as the Uterine Fibroid Symptoms Quality of Life, or UFS-QOL, discussed previously).

Alternative and complementary therapies are likely in the future to play an important role for fibroids in particular and gynecologic diseases in general. However, further testing needs to be conducted on all therapies to demonstrate which of them are safe and effective.

CHAPTER 23

What Can We Do about Fibroids?

It is unlikely that a "magic bullet" for fibroids will be found in my lifetime or in my daughter's reproductive years. My impression is that we will probably have many treatments for fibroids, since they are forming as a result of many different abnormalities. What will be important over the next decade is obtaining research funding to provide evidence-based medicine that will tell us which therapies are optimal for particular women or types of fibroids.

We also need advocacy. Lawmakers, doctors, and scientists need to know how much fibroids and the limitations of current therapies affect women's lives. I am aware of several efforts to increase their awareness of these issues. Congresswoman Stephanie Tubbs Jones and Senator Barbara Mikulski have introduced a bill in Congress called "The Uterine Fibroid Research and Education Act of 2005." This bill aims not only to provide increased funding for fibroid research but to educate women and health care providers about uterine fibroids. There are also two national organizations working in the field, the Fibroid Foundation (www.fibroidfoundation.org) and the National Uterine Fibroid Foundation (www.nuff.org). All these efforts should bring attention to the problem.

Given the high rate of fibroid recurrence, however, just developing new treatments will not be sufficient. We need to follow the same path that cardiovascular disease research has taken. Over my lifetime, instead of just aiming to better care for people who have heart attacks, research has brought us from better care to early intervention and then to prevention.

We continue to need scientific research to understand the molecular steps that lead to fibroid formation and the molecular steps that stimulate growth. Prevention has to be the strategy for the future. This is a difficult task, however, since the basic studies were not done 10 or 20 years ago that would make this field competitive for governmental and private research funds. Physicians, researchers, and patients must consider ways to bridge this funding and knowledge gap.

We also need clinical research to objectively test new treatments and optimize old ones. Again, this is a difficult task, since funding for studies is needed and both doctors and their patients must be willing to conduct and enroll in studies to determine outcomes.

Until then we have to make the best choices we can with intuition and careful consideration of the choices. I think of the choices for fibroid treatment as being part of a spectrum, as follows:

Watchful waiting
Medical treatment (birth control pills, Mirena IUD)
Focused ultrasound surgery
Hysteroscopic and laparoscopic myomectomy
Uterine artery embolization
Abdominal myomectomy
Hysterectomy

As you go down this list, the invasiveness of the procedure increases, and the time necessary for postoperative recovery increases. However, the certainty that you will get relief also increases. Fibroid recurrence is also an issue with any option other than hysterectomy.

Weighing these risks and benefits of therapy is a part of many fields of medicine today. Although some people argue that women should just accept hysterectomy, since it is a cost-effective, definitive solution, I believe this position represents an unfair bias for this disease. As I discussed in my presentation at the NIH International Congress called "Advances in Leiomyoma Research" (http://orwh.od.nih.gov/fibroid_conference/stewart.pdf), this is not the approach that has been taken in other diseases that affect quality of life. For example, for erectile dysfunction, a whole generation of surgical therapies were widely used before the development of new oral agents such as Viagra.

There are many factors that go into making decisions regarding treatment. The following checklist may be useful in helping you decide whether you need treatment and, if so, which treatment is best for you.

Do I need treatment?

1. Is heavy or prolonged menstrual bleeding a problem for me?
2. Is pelvic pressure and discomfort an issue for me?
3. Are there symptoms I have had so long that I am not even aware of them?
4. Am I planning a pregnancy in the near future?
5. If I wait, am I going to lose a minimally invasive option?
6. Are there any medical factors that complicate my decision making?

Once I have decided I need treatment:

1. Will solving the bleeding problem alone be enough?
2. Do I need resolution of the size- or "bulk"-related symptoms?
3. Do I need improvement in both?
4. How important is future pregnancy?
5. Do I want to optimize chances of pregnancy or just keep the door open?
6. Is keeping my uterus important to me even if I don't want pregnancy?
7. How many years do I likely have before menopause?
8. How important is it to me to not face the possibility of additional treatment in the future?
9. What are my work-related constraints?
10. Would I rather have a minimally invasive option that fails to adequately relieve my symptoms, or a more proven option that requires longer recovery?
11. Is having a flat stomach as important as solving the "bulk" symptoms?
12. Do I have other problems (such as abnormal Pap smears, endometriosis, adenomyosis, endometrial polyps, HLRCC syndrome, strong family history of ovarian cancer) that may be causing some of my symptoms or may make one treatment better than another for addressing both issues?

13. Which procedures does my doctor perform frequently?
14. Is it worth seeing an unfamiliar doctor or going to a less conveniently located hospital to have different options and, potentially, different outcomes?
15. Do I have any special medical conditions that would interfere with some treatments?

Appendix

Hints for Surgical Recovery

In this part of the book I share healing hints in the hope that they will help you recover and heal after surgery. Almost all the information that physicians can offer about how best to take care of yourself after surgery is based on what our patients tell us has worked for them. The information offered here is no different. I have learned what helps best from my patients (and from my own experience).

Pain Management

Many people try to do without pain medication following surgery. Although many of us are afraid of becoming addicted to pain medication, evidence suggests that there are indeed serious risks to *not* treating pain adequately. Recently hospital accreditation organizations have aggressively campaigned to get hospital personnel to assess and adequately treat pain in postoperative patients.[1]

The first rule of pain management is *to try to avoid pain*. That is why I like to use local anesthesia (anesthesia just like the dentist uses to numb gums) even for people who have general anesthesia and are "asleep" during surgery. I administer the local anesthetic even before I make my incision. This approach is called *preemptive analgesia*.[2] Scientific studies suggest that if the pain receptors are never stimulated, pain is better managed than if you provoke pain and then later try to treat the pain. A surgeon who handles the tissues gently during surgery also helps to decrease pain.

You cannot depend on the doctors or nurses to tell you when you need pain medication. You are more of an expert than they are, since only you know how much pain you are having. Most hospitals now use a simple pain scale for gauging pain, in which a score of 0 means that you have no pain and a score of 10 means you have the worst pain you can imagine. Most hospitals have a sign showing a series of face drawings in which the number 10 has a big frown or even tears and 0 has a big smile.

Pain after surgery is not like when you are at home and you have a slight headache and it may develop into a severe headache or it may disappear. After surgery, if you are uncomfortable now, you will be miserable in an hour. You need to anticipate where your pain is headed and ask for pain medication when your pain is a level 3 or 4 so it never gets to be an 8 or 9.

Intravenous pain medication may work within minutes, while oral pain medication can take significantly longer to work. The point is that pain medications do not work instantaneously, so it is better to ask for another dose of pain medication when you first become achy and uncomfortable rather than waiting until you are in severe pain. This is the key to not letting things get out of control.

The second rule of pain management is that *controlling pain is important for your physical recovery*. There are many things you need to do to optimize your surgical recovery, including coughing, rolling over in bed, and walking. If you have a pain level of 1 when you don't move and an 8 when you cough, you need more pain medication. I ask patients who tell me they are not in pain whether they can cough or roll over in bed without difficulty. Many of them say no. You may not notice the pain if you are able to lie perfectly still. However, because moving around after surgery is a key to avoiding postsurgical complications, you need to do normal everyday activities without hurting too much.

As more time elapses after your surgery, it can be difficult to recognize pain. Fatigue is a big problem following surgery, and we are not sure why it occurs. It seems reasonable, however, to believe that the body uses lots of metabolic energy to repair the damage of surgery. Low-level pain can be interpreted as fatigue, just as walking in uncomfortable shoes can be more tiring than when the shoes fit well. Sometimes fatigue improves with adequate pain relief.

Third, *it is often hard to provide perfect pain medication*, especially right after surgery. To get control of your pain, there may be times when you may feel goofy or tired or sleepy. On the other hand, you will be able to cough and roll over and move freely. Balancing the need for pain control and the ability to have a clear head is like walking a tightrope. You don't want to get too much or too little, but it is often hard to hit this absolute middle mark at all times. Although the goal is to minimize these swings to get relatively constant pain relief, you can also optimize your recovery by using them to your advantage. If you have just gotten pain medication and are comfortable, this is a good time to get up and walk. After walking, you will be tired as the pain medications reach maximal levels and begin to make you sleepy. This is a good time to nap.

Fourth, unless your doctor believes that certain pain medications are wrong for you, *often you will get optimal pain relief by combining different classes of drugs.* The same approach has been taken in anesthesia, so that, instead of having a walloping dose of a single medication to put you under, smaller amounts of different medications are used. The different medications work together (synergize) to give a greater effect than they could individually. The following types of medications can often be used for pain control postoperatively.

Narcotic Pain Medications

Narcotics are thought to be the strongest pain medications; available only by prescription, they generally are the most effective drugs for treating severe postoperative pain. Drugs in this category include Demerol, oxycodone, codeine, Dilaudid, and Vicodin. These agents are powerful pain medications that work on the brain. It is often necessary to take these drugs to get relief for severe pain in postoperative recovery, but they tend to cause nausea, constipation, and changes in thinking. People cannot drive or do highly skilled work when taking these medications. Long-term use can lead to tolerance and addiction, though these concerns generally are not appropriate when someone is using the drugs for relief of postsurgical pain.

Nonsteroidal Anti-inflammatory Agents

Nonsteroidal anti-inflammatory drugs (NSAIDs) are drugs that decrease the production of prostaglandins. Prostaglandins are compounds in the body that serve different functions and that are produced by the body as needed. Some prostaglandins are involved in transmitting nerve impulses; others cause inflammation. Blocking these prostaglandins helps control pain. There are prescription versions of NSAIDs, such as ibuprofen 400–800 mg and Anaprox 550 mg, and lower doses that are available over the counter, such as ibuprofen 200 mg and Aleve. These drugs are very effective in relieving muscular and inflammatory aches and pains. They can affect the function of blood platelets while they are being taken, and therefore they are not used after certain surgical procedures in which postoperative bleeding may be a problem. They can also cause stomach irritation and ulcers. They tend to have fewer side effects on the brain and on bowel habits and thus can complement narcotic pain medications (allowing for a lower dose of narcotics).

Acetaminophen

Acetaminophen (marketed as Tylenol) is a pain medication that can be used to augment either nonsteroidal or narcotic pain medication. Overdose on this medication can be very serious, however. Some of the narcotic pain medications come in formulations combining acetaminophen and narcotics in the same tablet. Percocet, for example, contains acetaminophen plus oxycodone. Before taking additional acetaminophen, you need to be sure that none of the other products you are taking contain acetaminophen. Under no circumstances should you take more than 4,000 mgs of acetaminophen in one day.

Agents for Neuropathic Pain

Agents for neuropathic pain include low-dose amitriptyline and gabapentin. These drugs are seldom prescribed after gynecologic surgery, but they are very useful in treating nerve-related (neuropathic) pain. The type of neuropathic pain most people have heard of is phantom limb pain, in which a person who has had an arm or leg removed still feels pain in that missing limb because of the continued firing of the nerves that used to direct that limb. Some reports suggest that nerve-related pain might be underreported in gynecologic patients.[3] Neuropathic pain produces specific symptoms following surgery: the pain is worse at night and feels like burning.[4] In addition, the slightest disturbance of the skin can lead to discomfort. Neuropathic pain may also be increased if you had an infection prior to surgery.

Dosages

Combining pain medications if there are no contraindications (reasons for *not* doing so) can be appropriate. For most of my postsurgical patients I combine nonsteroidal anti-inflammatory agents (NSAIDs) and narcotics. I add other agents if there are elements of continued pain or neuropathic pain.

After surgery, as soon as women are eating, it may be reasonable to take the NSAIDs with meals, which can provide baseline pain medication. Taking these drugs with meals also decreases the side effects of these drugs on the stomach. With a "base" of pain relief from a drug like ibuprofen at breakfast, lunch, and dinner, the amount of narcotics used is minimized, as well. (Acetaminophen can be used as baseline pain control for women unable to take NSAIDs.) Keeping a pain diary is easy and can be helpful, especially immediately after surgery, when you may be confused or tired when waking up in the middle of the night and may not be sure which pain medication is appropriate to take. The pain diary records your level of pain and your medication schedule.

With many pain medications it is possible to take less medication than is contained in one tablet. While one Percocet tablet may be appropriate for many people, some individuals get nausea and vomiting at this dose. Some individuals do perfectly well on 1/4 of a Percocet tablet every 3 hours; they would not be able to tolerate a whole tablet even twice a day. In general, taking smaller amounts more frequently may give you better pain relief than taking large amounts infrequently. You can check with your pharmacist to see whether the tablets you have can be safely divided. You should also let your doctor know if you are sensitive to medications and may need less than the standard amount.

Nausea

Nausea can be a major problem for some people following surgery. People who have "tender stomachs" and get carsick and airsick tend to have more problems with nausea after surgery. Other people have cast-iron stomachs and can wake up from anesthesia feeling as if they are ready for a cheeseburger. Sometimes it is hard to find out whether someone is nauseated because of too much pain or too much pain medication, since both situations can stimulate this feeling.

Again, *prevention is the first step*. If you have problems with nausea, let your anesthesiologist or anesthetist know about it prior to the surgery. The combination of medication used may be influenced by this information. Also, adjusting the amount or the route of pain medication, or both, may be helpful. Taking lower doses more frequently may help, since that schedule produces less variation in blood levels. The route of pain medication can also affect nausea; using a form that gets into the body much more slowly can help prevent nausea. Although patient-controlled anesthesia (in which the patient controls the amount of pain medication herself by using a pump that gives an intravenous dose) can be a great method for some people, for others the rapid increase in the blood level of narcotics provokes nausea, and the slower onset of a shot or a pill is desirable.

A number of excellent antinausea drugs are available now. When I first started my training, everyone receiving chemotherapy had terrible nausea and vomiting, and little could be done. Although some of the medications today cause sleepiness, severe nausea can be effectively treated.

Things to Pack for the Hospital

Most people know to bring a nightgown, robe, slippers, and basic toiletries with them to the hospital. The hospital will provide hospital gowns and basics such as a toothbrush and toothpaste, but once you are feeling better, you will want to use your own things. If you have sensitive skin, bringing your own pillowcase and sheet can be helpful. Hospital laundries may use detergents that you find irritating to your skin.

If you have critical medications you take regularly, you may want to place them in your bag. While you are in the hospital, you don't want to take anything without your doctor's approval. However, if your medication is not stocked in the hospital pharmacy (termed "on the formulary"), it may take a while to get it for you. For example, if you have migraines that really respond well to only one medication, your doctor may allow you to take your own if the hospital does not stock this medication.

It is also nice to have something to do when you feel bored. Generally people don't have a long enough attention span for reading a book following surgery, but magazines or listening to books on tape or CD can be relaxing. Also some sort of private music player (iPod or CD player) can help you relax. Generally it needs to be used with an earphone so as not to disturb other patients.

Finally, it is worth having a few dollars with you, in case you want a newspaper or magazine. Also, once you are able to eat an unrestricted diet, with the approval of your nurses, you may find the food sold in the hospital lobby to visitors more appetizing than what is served to you in your room.

Preparing Your Home for Your Return from Surgery

Most people worry about getting up and down stairs in their house or apartment following surgery, but most patients are able to go up and down stairs, even on their first or second postoperative days. Many people, however, feel more comfortable putting both feet on every step before continuing, like a toddler. This technique minimizes use of the abdominal muscles following abdominal surgery. Rarely, people will decide to sit down and move on their bottom up the steps instead of walking. Because most people have limited stamina after the surgery, minimizing the number of trips up and down the steps is appropriate.

Having someone who is able to bring things to you can be useful after surgery! A small bell can be used to summon someone for help if necessary and can be especially welcome if you have small children at home who would be glad to help by getting the newspaper or a box of tissues.

It is often helpful to have a number of specific items on a bedside table. In addition to a light and a clock, you should have room for your medication and a glass of water. It is also helpful to have a small snack like crackers so that you don't have to take pain medication on an empty stomach. A pad or paper to write on and a pen can be useful, especially because people tend to be more forgetful when they are taking pain medication; writing things down as you think of them means you will not forget them.

It is best to move the phone off the bedside table, or at least turn the ringer off, so you don't feel compelled to answer it. When you are recovering from surgery, you should talk only to the people you want to talk to and only when you want to.

Bathroom Safety

Most women can take a shower shortly after surgery, although a bath may be contraindicated for up to 2 weeks. Water does not seep into the abdomen during a shower, but if you are sitting under 6 inches of water, it might. Placing a chair in or near the bathroom is a good idea. Often after taking a hot shower, you may feel woozy and will need to sit down as you dry yourself or prepare to get dressed. Since some stretching is usually easier than bending over for people with abdominal incisions, placing soap and shampoo on a rack over the showerhead can be easier than reaching down to the tub to retrieve these items.

Bowel and Bladder Concerns

Constipation can be a problem following surgery and is often related to the narcotic pain medications. These medications slow down the motility of the intestinal tract. That plus the decreased activity and tendency to eat bland food contributes to substantial bowel problems for some, but not all, people. Most women need at least some narcotic pain medication following surgery, however, so doing without is not usually an option.

Increasing movement, especially walking, is always helpful in stimulating the bowels. Most women who have had an abdominal or vaginal incision worry about straining or contracting their abdominal muscles when they have a bowel movement. People are afraid of having their incision split open, but this almost never happens. Fear of hurting the incision can lead to even more constipation.

Increasing the amount of fruit and vegetables or other kinds of fiber in the diet can also help overcome constipation. Some people find using a stool softener such as Colace helpful. Generally, however, you should not use a laxative without discussing it with your doctor.

Severe diarrhea is also something that you should report to your doctor in the postoperative period. While diarrhea could be related to food you have eaten, there are rare instances when it is a sign of a postoperative complication. Sometimes your doctor will need you to bring in a stool sample to look for a specific toxin (*Clostridium difficile*) that can develop in a person treated with antibiotics (most women undergoing gynecologic surgery will get preoperative antibiotics). Other times you will be asked to come in for a physical exam because diarrhea can be a symptom of major bowel problems following surgery. It is most important to report diarrhea if you also have other symptoms including a fever, nausea, vomiting, or blood in your stool.

Many procedures require that the bladder be emptied during surgery. The most common way to do this is to place a Foley catheter in the bladder. A Foley is a hollow tube connected to a bag to collect urine. Near the tip inside the bladder there is a small balloon to keep the catheter from falling out of the bladder. This is why the catheter needs to be removed by a medical professional: the balloon must be deflated first.

After many major surgeries the Foley is kept in the bladder overnight. There are two reasons for this: first, it means you don't have to get up and go to the bathroom right away. Second, it allows the medical staff to measure more easily and accurately the amount of urine you are making, which can be important to be certain you are not having bleeding or fluid problems.

Once the catheter is taken out, it takes a while for your bladder to fill and for you to feel the need to go. Peeing the first time after taking out the catheter is usually uncomfortable, and the discomfort may continue during the next couple of times. It can feel as if the catheter is still in or the urethral opening is raw and sore. This is normal. If the discomfort gets worse rather than better over the first day or two, however, you may need to have your doctors check for a bladder infection, which can occur after having a catheter in place. It is also important to feel that you are emptying your bladder. Sometimes after surgery you can "go" but not fully empty it. An ultrasound machine can measure the amount of urine remaining in your bladder and help determine whether your bladder needs additional rest.

Movement

Particularly for women with large fibroids, a certain amount of muscular reprogramming may need to take place following a hysterectomy or myomectomy. Having 2 pounds of fibroids resting on your spine and legs causes your body to adapt in much the same way that your shoulders adapt to carrying a heavy load in a backpack. Furthermore, since the fibroid uterus can be asymmetrical, the load can be distributed so the stress is different in each leg and on different parts of the spine. The same thing can be seen when a woman always carries a heavy purse or briefcase on the same shoulder, making one shoulder higher than the other because of muscular contraction. Some women benefit from physical therapy or supervised exercise following surgery. There is some recent evidence that some of the things people do all the time after surgery—like getting up out of a chair—put as much strain on the abdominal cavity as what we think of as more vigorous exercise.[5]

One of the hardest things to do after abdominal surgery is getting into and out of bed. Hospital beds typically have a back that rolls up, which makes the task easier. Once you get home, however, getting out of bed can be a major challenge. Some people find that lying on their stomach and moving their legs off the bed is a better strategy than trying to sit up. Placing your feet on the floor and straightening your back is often easier on your abdominal muscles than doing a sit-up-like motion.

Walking is often the ideal exercise for those early days at home. It is best to walk in a somewhat circular path so that you do not get too far from your home before getting tired and to set a goal of walking a little farther every day.

Generally, vigorously using muscles in the abdomen, particularly the rectus muscles (the muscles used in sit-ups), is contraindicated for the 6 weeks after abdominal surgery. Heat and stretching that does not bother the stomach muscles can be helpful for surgical recovery. Gentle yoga can be beneficial for postoperative recovery. Even though your doctor may tell you not to employ these techniques near your incision, often it is other muscles that become strained and sore. In trying to protect the abdominal muscles, people often move in a way that makes the shoulders and back uncomfortable.

Massage can be useful following surgery. A general relaxation massage can help relax all the muscles you are overusing, like the shoulders and the back. Also, once the incision is closed, usually after about 10 days, massaging the incision can be helpful. Not only does it feel pleasant, but it may also increase the blood flow to the tissue and break up collagen fibers that can form and cause scar tissue. Although some people recommend using particular massage oils, such as vitamin E oil, other studies suggest that the physical action of massage is more important than the type of oil or cream.

Driving

Rather than designating a specific time when driving can be resumed, I recommend that you ask yourself three questions:

Am I off all narcotic pain medications?

Could I slam on the brakes without problem?

Do I have the energy to drive there, do what I need to do, and drive home again?

Unless you can answer yes to all three of these questions, you are not ready to drive. Additionally I recommend that the first few times you drive you take a responsible second driver with you. We all overestimate what we can do, and it is embarrassing to ask someone to come pick you up after a quick trip to the grocery store. On your first trip out, it's common to be too tired to even wait at the checkout line. You will instead drive home, even if you are exhausted. However, if you have a friend or relative along, it is easy to say, "Gee, would you mind driving home?" And as with walking, gradually increase the length of your driving trips as your recovery progresses.

Protecting Your Emotional Health

Many people find they are uncomfortable mentally while recovering from surgery. Not only is your stamina decreased, but your attention span may be affected by the pain medication. Television is a solution many of us utilize, but at some point it becomes overwhelming. Books on tape can be a good solution, as can simple puzzles or handwork such as knitting or crocheting.

For women, especially mothers, who are used to caring for everyone else, the tendency is to tell everyone that you are fine and doing well after surgery. Even if you think you are doing fine, you will benefit from accepting help during these times. Having others cook and bring by food is a great boon during recovery. Also, try to learn to feel comfortable letting some things go by the wayside while you are recovering. Using paper plates instead of washing dishes, and using wash-dry-fold services at the Laundromat, may be helpful.

Surgical Menopause

Rarely do the ovaries have to be removed at the time of fibroid surgery, but for some women they do, and these women may find that having a sudden surgical menopause and postoperative recovery at the same time can be too much. This can be especially true for younger women who have not started the menopausal transition and who go overnight from having normal estrogen levels to menopausal levels of estrogen. In this group of women I still sometimes see patients who (often reluctantly) report crying uncontrollably or feeling like their brain is not working normally. We do know that estrogen has real effects on the brain, but we don't know how to control this problem following surgical removal of the ovaries. I suspect that these are common problems for women following oophorectomy (loss of their ovaries), but women are too embarrassed to discuss these problems with their doctors.

For this reason I often recommend to women having their ovaries removed that they use an estrogen patch during their postoperative recovery. You want to use the patch rather than a pill, since the combination of having surgery and taking oral estrogens increases the risk of major blood clots in the legs and lungs. If things go smoothly, you can rapidly taper the dose of estrogen after your postoperative visit. That way you deal with surgical recovery and menopausal changes at different times, since dealing with both simultaneously can be overwhelming.

Doses required for hormone therapy in this situation may be higher than doses required with regular menopausal hormone therapy (see Chapter 13). Also, women who have had a hysterectomy are able to take estrogen alone rather than an estrogen-progestin combination, and studies suggest this regimen has fewer long-term risks.

References

Introduction

1. Angier N. *Woman: An Intimate Geography.* New York: Random House, 1999.
2. Harden T. "Diagnosing fibroids is simple; Deciding what to do is hard." *New York Times.* June 13, 1999: 14.

Chapter 1. Who Gets Fibroids, and What Are the Symptoms?

1. Garcia CR, Tureck RW. Submucosal leiomyomas and infertility. *Fertility and Sterility.* 1984;42(1):16–19.
2. Pritts EA. Fibroids and infertility: a systematic review of the evidence. *Obstetrical and Gynecological Survey.* Aug 2001;56(8):483–491.
3. Cramer SF, Patel A. The frequency of uterine leiomyomas. *American Journal of Clinical Pathology.* 1990;94(4):435–438.
4. Marshall LM, Spiegelman D, Barbieri RL, et al. Variation in the incidence of uterine leiomyoma among premenopausal women by age and race. *Obstetrics and Gynecology.* 1997;90(6):967–973.
5. Kjerulff KH, Langenberg P, Seidman JD, et al. Uterine leiomyomas: racial differences in severity, symptoms and age at diagnosis. *Journal of Reproductive Medicine.* 1996;41(7):483–490.
6. Baird D, Dunson D, Hill M, et al. High cumulative incidence of uterine leiomyoma in black and white women: ultrasound evidence. *American Journal of Obstetrics and Gynecology.* 2003;188(1):100–107.
7. Marshall LM, Spiegelman D, Manson JE, et al. Risk of uterine leiomyomata among premenopausal women in relation to body size and cigarette smoking. *Epidemiology.* 1998;9(5):511–517.
8. Vikhlyaeva EM, Khodzhaeva ZS, Fantschenko ND. Familial predisposition to uterine leiomyomas. *International Journal of Gynaecology and Obstetrics.* Nov 1995;51(2):127–131.
9. Van Voorhis BJ, Romitti PA, Jones MP. Family history as a risk factor for development of uterine leiomyomas. Results of a pilot study. *Journal of Reproductive Medicine.* Aug 2002;47(8):663–669.

10. Ross RK, Pike MC, Vessey MP, et al. Risk factors for uterine fibroids: reduced risk associated with oral contraceptives. *British Medical Journal* (Clinical Research ed.). 1986;293(6543):359–362.

11. Parazzini F, La Vecchia C, Negri E, et al. Epidemiologic characteristics of women with uterine fibroids: a case-control study. *Obstetrics and Gynecology.* 1988;72(6):853–857.

12. Wise LA, Palmer JR, Harlow BL, et al. Reproductive factors, hormonal contraception, and risk of uterine leiomyomata in African-American women: a prospective study. *American Journal of Epidemiology.* Jan 15 2004;159(2): 113–123.

13. Cesen-Cummings K, Copland JA, Barrett JC, et al. Pregnancy, parturition, and prostaglandins: defining uterine leiomyomas. *Environmental Health Perspectives.* 2000;108 Suppl 5:817–820.

14. Chiaffarino F, Parazzini F, La Vecchia C, et al. Use of oral contraceptives and uterine fibroids: results from a case-control study. *British Journal of Obstetrics and Gynaecology.* 1999;106(8):857–860.

15. Marshall LM, Spiegelman D, Goldman MB, et al. A prospective study of reproductive factors and oral contraceptive use in relation to the risk of uterine leiomyomata. *Fertility and Sterility.* 1998;70(3):432–439.

16. Parazzini F, Negri E, La Vecchia C, et al. Uterine myomas and smoking. Results from an Italian study. *Journal of Reproductive Medicine.* 1996;41(5): 316–320.

17. Faerstein E, Szklo M, Rosenshein N. Risk factors for uterine leiomyoma: a practice-based case-control study. I. African-American heritage, reproductive history, body size, and smoking. *American Journal of Epidemiology.* 2001;153(1):1–10.

18. Chiaffarino F, Parazzini F, La Vecchia C, et al. Diet and uterine myomas. *Obstetrics and Gynecology.* 1999;94(3):395–398.

19. Wise LA, Palmer JR, Harlow BL, et al. Risk of uterine leiomyomata in relation to tobacco, alcohol and caffeine consumption in the Black Women's Health Study. *American Journal of Physiology.* Aug 2004;19(8):1746–1754.

20. Sato F, Nishi M, Kudo R, Miyake H. Body fat distribution and uterine leiomyomas. *Journal of Epidemiology.* Aug 1998;8(3):176–180.

Chapter 2. What Are Uterine Fibroids?

1. Andersen J, DyReyes VM, Barbieri RL, et al. Leiomyoma primary cultures have elevated transcriptional response to estrogen compared with autologous myometrial cultures. *Journal of the Society for Gynecologic Investigation.* 1995;2(3):542–551.

2. Linder D, Gartler SM. Glucose-6-phosphate dehydrogenase mosaicism: utilization as a cell marker in the study of leiomyomas. *Science.* 1965;150(692): 67–69.

3. Mashal RD, Fejzo ML, Friedman AJ, et al. Analysis of androgen receptor DNA reveals the independent clonal origins of uterine leiomyomata and the secondary nature of cytogenetic aberrations in the development of leiomyomata. *Genes, Chromosomes and Cancer.* 1994;11(1):1–6.

4. Cramer SF, Patel A. The frequency of uterine leiomyomas. *American Journal of Clinical Pathology.* 1990;94(4):435–438.
5. Oelsner G, Elizur SE, Frenkel Y, Carp H. Giant uterine tumors: two cases with different clinical presentations. *Obstetrics and Gynecology.* May 2003; 101(5 Pt 2):1088–1091.
6. Wamsteker K, Emanuel MH, de Kruif JH. Transcervical hysteroscopic resection of submucous fibroids for abnormal uterine bleeding: results regarding the degree of intramural extension. *Obstetrics and Gynecology.* Nov 1993;82(5):736–740.
7. Stewart EA, Friedman AJ, Peck K, Nowak RA. Relative overexpression of collagen type I and collagen type III messenger ribonucleic acids by uterine leiomyomas during the proliferative phase of the menstrual cycle. *Journal of Clinical Endocrinology and Metabolism.* 1994;79(3):900–906.
8. Stewart EA, Nowak RA. New concepts in the treatment of uterine leiomyomas. *Obstetrics and Gynecology.* 1998;92:624–627.
9. Patterson-Keels LM, Selvaggi SM, Haefner HK, Randolph JF, Jr. Morphologic assessment of endometrium overlying submucosal leiomyomas. *Journal of Reproductive Medicine.* 1994;39(8):579–584.
10. Anania CA, Stewart EA, Quade BJ, et al. Expression of the fibroblast growth factor receptor in women with leiomyomas and abnormal uterine bleeding. *Molecular Human Reproduction.* 1997;3(8):685–691.

Chapter 3. Why We Are So Far Behind in Understanding and Treating Fibroids

1. Levy D, Brink S. *A Change of Heart.* New York: Alfred A. Knopf, 2005.
2. Savage DG, Antman KH. Imatinib mesylate—a new oral targeted therapy. *New England Journal of Medicine.* Feb 28 2002;346(9):683–693.
3. Van de Vijver MJ, He YD, van't Veer LJ, et al. A gene-expression signature as a predictor of survival in breast cancer. *New England Journal of Medicine.* Dec 19 2002;347(25):1999–2009.
4. Flynn M, Jamison M, Datta S, Myers E. Health care resource use for uterine fibroid tumors in the United States. *American Journal of Obstetrics and Gynecology.* Oct 2006;195(4):955–964.
5. Hartmann KE, Birnbaum H, Ben-Hamadi R, et al. Annual costs associated with diagnosis of uterine leiomyomata. *Obstetrics and Gynecology.* Oct 2006;108(4):930–937.

Chapter 4. The Endocrinology of the Uterus

1. Irwin KL, Weiss NS, Lee NC, Peterson HB. Tubal sterilization, hysterectomy, and the subsequent occurrence of epithelial ovarian cancer. *American Journal of Epidemiology.* 1991;134(4):362–369.
2. Hankinson SE, Hunter DJ, Colditz GA, et al. Tubal ligation, hysterectomy, and risk of ovarian cancer. A prospective study. *JAMA: Journal of the American Medical Association.* 1993;270(23):2813–2818.
3. Chwalisz K, DeManno D, Garg R, et al. Therapeutic potential for the selective progesterone receptor modulator asoprisnil in the treatment of leiomyomata. *Seminars in Reproductive Medicine.* May 2004;22(2):113–119.

194   REFERENCES

4. Chwalisz K, Perez MC, Demanno D, et al. Selective progesterone receptor modulator development and use in the treatment of leiomyomata and endometriosis. *Endocrine Reviews.* May 2005;26(3):423–438.
5. Pedeutour F, Quade BJ, Weremowicz S, et al. Localization and expression of the human estrogen receptor beta gene in uterine leiomyomata. *Genes, Chromosomes and Cancer.* 1998;23(4):361–366.
6. Benassayag C, Leroy MJ, Rigourd V, et al. Estrogen receptors (ERalpha/ERbeta) in normal and pathological growth of the human myometrium: pregnancy and leiomyoma. *American Journal of Physiology.* 1999;276(6 Pt 1):E1112–1118.
7. Stewart EA, Austin DJ, Jain P, et al. RU486 suppresses prolactin production in explant cultures of leiomyoma and myometrium. *Fertility and Sterility.* 1996;65(6):1119–1124.
8. Mangrulkar RS, Ono M, Ishikawa M, et al. Isolation and characterization of heparin-binding growth factors in human leiomyomas and normal myometrium. *Biology of Reproduction.* 1995;53(3):636–646.
9. Anania CA, Stewart EA, Quade BJ, et al. Expression of the fibroblast growth factor receptor in women with leiomyomas and abnormal uterine bleeding. *Molecular Human Reproduction.* 1997;3(8):685–691.
10. Chegini N, Zhao Y, Williams RS, Flanders KC. Human uterine tissue throughout the menstrual cycle expresses transforming growth factor-beta 1 (TGF beta 1), TGF beta 2, TGF beta 3, and TGF beta type II receptor messenger ribonucleic acid and protein and contains [125I]TGF beta 1–binding sites. *Endocrinology.* 1994;135(1):439–449.
11. Lee BS, Nowak RA. Human leiomyoma smooth muscle cells show increased expression of transforming growth factor-beta 3 (TGF beta 3) and altered responses to the antiproliferative effects of TGF beta. *Journal of Clinical Endocrinology and Metabolism.* 2001;86(2):913–920.
12. Sozen I, Arici A. Interactions of cytokines, growth factors, and the extracellular matrix in the cellular biology of uterine leiomyomata. *Fertility and Sterility.* 2002;78(1):1–12.
13. Dou Q, Tarnuzzer RW, Williams RS, et al. Differential expression of matrix metalloproteinases and their tissue inhibitors in leiomyomata: a mechanism for gonadotrophin releasing hormone agonist–induced tumour regression. *Molecular Human Reproduction.* 1997;3(11):1005–1014.
14. Palmer SS, Haynes-Johnson D, Diehl T, Nowak RA. Increased expression of stromelysin 3 mRNA in leiomyomas (uterine fibroids) compared with myometrium. *Journal of the Society for Gynecologic Investigation.* 1998;5(4):203–209.
15. Chegini N, Luo X, Ding L, Ripley D. The expression of Smads and transforming growth factor beta receptors in leiomyoma and myometrium and the effect of gonadotropin releasing hormone analogue therapy. *Molecular and Cellular Endocrinology.* Nov 14 2003;209(1–2):9–16.
16. Stewart EA, Friedman AJ, Peck K, Nowak RA. Relative overexpression of collagen type I and collagen type III messenger ribonucleic acids by uterine leiomyomas during the proliferative phase of the menstrual cycle. *Journal of Clinical Endocrinology and Metabolism.* 1994;79(3):900–906.

17. Catherino WH, Leppert PC, Stenmark MH, et al. Reduced dermatopontin expression is a molecular link between uterine leiomyomas and keloids. *Genes, Chromosomes and Cancer.* Jul 2004;40(3):204–217.
18. Rein MS, Friedman AJ, Pandian MR, Heffner LJ. The secretion of insulin-like growth factors I and II by explant cultures of fibroids and myometrium from women treated with a gonadotropin-releasing hormone agonist. *Obstetrics and Gynecology.* 1990;76(3 Pt 1):388–394.
19. Giudice LC, Irwin JC, Dsupin BA, et al. Insulin-like growth factor (IGF), IGF binding protein (IGFBP), and IGF receptor gene expression and IGFBP synthesis in human uterine leiomyomata. *Human Reproduction.* 1993;8(11): 1796–1806.
20. Burroughs KD, Howe SR, Okubo Y, et al. Dysregulation of IGF-I signaling in uterine leiomyoma. *Journal of Endocrinology.* Jan 2002;172(1):83–93.

Chapter 5. Why Do Fibroids Form?

1. Stewart EA, Nowak RA. New concepts in the treatment of uterine leiomyomas. *Obstetrics and Gynecology* 1998; 92:624–627.
2. Nowak R. Indentification of new therapies for leiomyomas: what in vitro studies can tell us. *Clinical Obstetrics and Gynecology* 2001; 44:327–334.
3. Sampson JA. The blood supply of uterine myomata. *Surgery, Gynecology and Obstetrics.* 1912;14:215–230.
4. Farrer-Brown G, Beilby JO, Tarbit MH. Venous changes in the endometrium of myomatous uteri. *Obstetrics and Gynecology.* 1971;38(5):743–751.
5. Mangrulkar RS, Ono M, Ishikawa M, et al. Isolation and characterization of heparin-binding growth factors in human leiomyomas and normal myometrium. *Biology of Reproduction* 1995; 53:636–646.
6. Buttram VC, Jr., Reiter RC. Uterine leiomyomata: etiology, symptomatology, and management. *Fertility and Sterility.* 1981;36(4):433–445.
7. Stewart EA, Nowak RA. Leiomyoma-related bleeding: a classic hypothesis updated for the molecular era. *Human Reproduction Update.* 1996;2(4):295–306.
8. Coutinho E, Segal S. *Is Menstruation Obsolete?* New York: Oxford University Press, 1999.
9. Andersen J, Barbieri RL. Abnormal gene expression in uterine leiomyomas. *Journal of the Society for Gynecologic Investigation* 1995; 2:663–672.
10. Stewart EA, Floor AE, Jain P, Nowak RA. Increased expression of messenger RNA for collagen type I, collagen type III, and fibronectin in myometrium of pregnancy. *Obstetrics and Gynecology* 1995; 86:417–422.
11. Cesen-Cummings K, Copland JA, Barrett JC, et al. Pregnancy, parturition, and prostaglandins: defining uterine leiomyomas. *Environmental Health Perspectives* 2000; 108 Suppl 5:817–820.

Chapter 6. Diagnosis

1. Goldstein SR, Zeltser I, Horan CK, et al. Ultrasonography-based triage for perimenopausal patients with abnormal uterine bleeding. *American Journal of Obstetrics and Gynecology.* Jul 1997;177(1):102–108.

2. Breitkopf D, Goldstein SR, Seeds JW. ACOG technology assessment in obstetrics and gynecology. Number 3, September 2003. Saline infusion sonohysterography. *Obstetrics and Gynecology.* Sep 2003;102(3):659–662.
3. Towbin NA, Gviazda IM, March CM. Office hysteroscopy versus transvaginal ultrasonography in the evaluation of patients with excessive uterine bleeding. *American Journal of Obstetrics and Gynecology.* 1996;174(6):1678–1682.
4. Schwartz LB, Zawin M, Carcangiu ML, et al. Does pelvic magnetic resonance imaging differentiate among the histologic subtypes of uterine leiomyomata? *Fertility and Sterility.* 1998;70(3):580–587.
5. Kyei-Mensah A, Maconochie N, Zaidi J, et al. Transvaginal three-dimensional ultrasound: reproducibility of ovarian and endometrial volume measurements. *Fertility and Sterility.* Nov 1996;66(5):718–722.
6. La Torre R, De Felice C, De Angelis C, et al. Transvaginal sonographic evaluation of endometrial polyps: a comparison with two dimensional and three dimensional contrast sonography. *Clinical and Experimental Obstetrics and Gynecology.* 1999;26(3–4):171–173.
7. Stewart EA, Faur AV, Wise LA, et al. Predictors of subsequent surgery for uterine leiomyomata after abdominal myomectomy. *Obstetrics and Gynecology.* 2002;99(3):426–432.
8. Kouides PA, Conard J, Peyvandi F, et al. Hemostasis and menstruation: appropriate investigation for underlying disorders of hemostasis in women with excessive menstrual bleeding. *Fertility and Sterility.* Nov 2005;84(5):1345–1351.
9. Lukes AS, Kadir RA, Peyvandi F, Kouides PA. Disorders of hemostasis and excessive menstrual bleeding: prevalence and clinical impact. *Fertility and Sterility.* Nov 2005;84(5):1338–1344.

Chapter 7. When Fibroids Come Back

1. Malone LJ. Myomectomy: recurrence after removal of solitary and multiple myomas. *Obstetrics and Gynecology.* 1969;34(2):200–203.
2. Candiani GB, Fedele L, Parazzini F, Villa L. Risk of recurrence after myomectomy. *British Journal of Obstetrics and Gynaecology.* 1991;98(4):385–389.
3. Fedele L, Parazzini F, Luchini L, et al. Recurrence of fibroids after myomectomy: a transvaginal ultrasonographic study. *Human Reproduction.* 1995;10(7):1795–1796.
4. Acien P, Quereda F. Abdominal myomectomy: results of a simple operative technique. *Fertility and Sterility.* 1996;65(1):41–51.
5. Stewart EA, Faur AV, Wise LA, et al. Predictors of subsequent surgery for uterine leiomyomata after abdominal myomectomy. *Obstetrics and Gynecology.* 2002;99(3):426–432.
6. *Surgical alternatives to hysterectomy in the management of leiomyomas.* Practice Bulletin Vol No. 16: American College of Obstetricians and Gynecologists; 2000.
7. Rein MS, Powell WL, Walters FC, et al. Cytogenetic abnormalities in uterine myomas are associated with myoma size. *Molecular Human Reproduction.* 1998;4(1):83–86.

8. Hanafi M. Predictors of leiomyoma recurrence after myomectomy. *Obstetrics and Gynecology.* 2005;105(4):877–881.
9. Zhou X, Benson KF, Ashar HR, Chada K. Mutation responsible for the mouse pygmy phenotype in the developmentally regulated factor HMGI-C. *Nature.* 1995;376(6543):771–774.
10. Schoenberg Fejzo M, Ashar HR, Krauter KS, et al. Translocation breakpoints upstream of the HMGIC gene in uterine leiomyomata suggest dysregulation of this gene by a mechanism different from that in lipomas. *Genes, Chromosomes and Cancer.* 1996;17(1):1–6.

Chapter 8. Surgery Inside the Uterus

1. Wamsteker K, Emanuel MH, de Kruif JH. Transcervical hysteroscopic resection of submucous fibroids for abnormal uterine bleeding: results regarding the degree of intramural extension. *Obstetrics and Gynecology.* Nov 1993;82 (5):736–740.
2. Isaacson KB. Complications of hysteroscopy. *Obstetrics and Gynecology Clinics of North America.* Mar 1999;26(1):39–51.
3. Kim AH, Keltz MD, Arici A, et al. Dilutional hyponatremia during hysteroscopic myomectomy with sorbitol-mannitol distention medium. *Journal of the American Association of Gynecologic Laparoscopists.* 1995;2(2):237–242.
4. Emanuel MH, Wamsteker K. The intra uterine morcellator: a new hysteroscopic operating technique to remove intrauterine polyps and myomas. *Journal of Minimally Invasive Gynecology.* Jan–Feb 2005;12(1):62–66.
5. Emanuel MH, Wamsteker K, Lammes FB. Is dilatation and curettage obsolete for diagnosing intrauterine disorders in premenopausal patients with persistent abnormal uterine bleeding? *Acta Obstetricia et Gynecologica Scandinavica.* Jan 1997;76(1):65–68.
6. Rogerson L, Duffy S, Crocombe W, et al. Management of menorrhagia— SMART study (Satisfaction with Mirena and Ablation: a Randomised Trial). *BJOG: An International Journal of Obstetrics and Gynaecology* Oct 2000; 107(10):1325–1326.
7. Mercorio F, De Simone R, Di Spiezio Sardo A, et al. The effect of a levonorgestrel-releasing intrauterine device in the treatment of myoma-related menorrhagia. *Contraception.* Apr 2003;67(4):277–280.

Chapter 9. Laparoscopic Myomectomy and Myolysis

1. Dubuisson J, Chapron C, Levy L. Difficulties and complications of laparoscopic myomectomy. *Journal of Gynecologic Surgery.* 1996;12(3):159–165.
2. Goldfarb HA. Bipolar laparoscopic needles for myoma coagulation. *Journal of the American Association of Gynecologic Laparoscopists.* 1995;2(2):175–179.
3. Stewart EA, Liau AS, Friedman AJ. Operative laparoscopy followed by colpotomy for resecting a colonic leiomyosarcoma. A case report. *Journal of Reproductive Medicine.* 1991;36(12):883–884.
4. Advincula AP, Song A, Burke W, Reynolds RK. Preliminary experience with robot-assisted laparoscopic myomectomy. *Journal of the American Association of Gynecologic Laparoscopists.* Nov 2004;11(4):511–518.

198   REFERENCES

5. Nezhat C. The "cons" of laparoscopic myomectomy in women who may reproduce in the future. *International Journal of Fertility and Menopausal Studies.* 1996;41(3):280–283.
6. Harris WJ. Uterine dehiscence following laparoscopic myomectomy. *Obstetrics and Gynecology.* 1992;80(3 Pt 2):545–546.
7. Arcangeli S, Pasquarette MM. Gravid uterine rupture after myolysis. *Obstetrics and Gynecology.* 1997;89(5 Pt 2):857.
8. Pelosi MA, III, Pelosi MA. Spontaneous uterine rupture at thirty-three weeks subsequent to previous superficial laparoscopic myomectomy. *American Journal of Obstetrics and Gynecology.* 1997;177(6):1547–1549.
9. Hockstein S. Spontaneous uterine rupture in the early third trimester after laparoscopically assisted myomectomy. A case report. *Journal of Reproductive Medicine.* 2000;45(2):139–141.
10. Landi S, Fiaccavento A, Zaccoletti R, et al. Pregnancy outcomes and deliveries after laparoscopic myomectomy. *Journal of the American Association of Gynecologic Laparoscopists.* May 2003;10(2):177–181.
11. Malzoni M, Rotond M, Perone C, et al. Fertility after laparoscopic myomectomy of large uterine myomas: operative technique and preliminary results. *European Journal of Gynaecological Oncology.* 2003;24(1):79–82.

Chapter 10. Abdominal Myomectomy

1. LaMorte AI, Lalwani S, Diamond MP. Morbidity associated with abdominal myomectomy. *Obstetrics and Gynecology.* 1993;82(6):897–900.
2. Ecker JL, Foster JT, Friedman AJ. Abdominal hysterectomy or abdominal myomectomy for symptomatic leiomyoma: a comparison of preoperative demography and postoperative morbidity. *Journal of Gynecologic Surgery.* 1995;11(1):11–18.
3. Iverson RE, Jr., Chelmow D, Strohbehn K, et al. Relative morbidity of abdominal hysterectomy and myomectomy for management of uterine leiomyomas. *Obstetrics and Gynecology.* 1996;88(3):415–419.
4. Ginsburg ES, Benson CB, Garfield JM, et al. The effect of operative technique and uterine size on blood loss during myomectomy: a prospective randomized study. *Fertility and Sterility.* 1993;60(6):956–962.
5. Frederick J, Fletcher H, Simeon D, et al. Intramyometrial vasopressin as a haemostatic agent during myomectomy. *British Journal of Obstetrics and Gynaecology.* 1994;101(5):435–437.
6. Fletcher H, Frederick J, Hardie M, Simeon D. A randomized comparison of vasopressin and tourniquet as hemostatic agents during myomectomy. *Obstetrics and Gynecology.* 1996;87(6):1014–1018.
7. Hutchins FL, Jr. A randomized comparison of vasopressin and tourniquet as hemostatic agents during myomectomy. *Obstetrics and Gynecology.* 1996;88(4 Pt 1):639–640.
8. Garnet JD. Uterine rupture during pregnancy. *Obstetrics and Gynecology.* 1964;23:898–905.

Chapter 11. Uterine Artery Embolization

1. Ravina JH, Herbreteau D, Ciraru-Vigneron N, et al. Arterial embolisation to treat uterine myomata. *Lancet.* 1995;346(8976):671–672.
2. Goodwin SC, Walker WJ. Uterine artery embolization for the treatment of uterine fibroids. *Current Opinion in Obstetrics and Gynecology.* 1998;10(4): 315–320.
3. Spies JB, Ascher SA, Roth AR, et al. Uterine artery embolization for leiomyomata. *Obstetrics and Gynecology.* 2001;98(1):29–34.
4. Stewart E. Nonsurgical treatment of uterine fibroids. *Infertility and Reproductive Medical Clinics of North America.* 2002;13:393–405.
5. Worthington-Kirsch R, Spies JB, Myers ER, et al. The Fibroid Registry for outcomes data (FIBROID) for uterine embolization: short-term outcomes. *Obstetrics and Gynecology.* Jul 2005;106(1):52–59.
6. Yeagley TJ, Goldberg J, Klein TA, Bonn J. Labial necrosis after uterine artery embolization for leiomyomata. *Obstetrics and Gynecology.* 2002;100(5 Pt 1):881–882.
7. Dietz DM, Stahlfeld KR, Bansal SK, Christopherson WA. Buttock necrosis after uterine artery embolization. *Obstetrics and Gynecology.* Nov 2004;104 (5 Pt 2):1159–1161.
8. Spies JB, Spector A, Roth AR, et al. Complications after uterine artery embolization for leiomyomas. *Obstetrics and Gynecology.* 2002;100(5 Pt 1):873–880.
9. Pron G, Mocarski E, Bennett J, et al. Tolerance, hospital stay, and recovery after uterine artery embolization for fibroids: the Ontario Uterine Fibroid Embolization Trial. *Journal of Vascular and Interventional Radiology.* Oct 2003;14(10):1243–1250.
10. DeSouza N, Williams A. Uterine arterial embolization for leiomyomas: perfusion and volume changes at MR imaging and relation to clinical outcome. *Radiology.* 2002;222:367–374.
11. Spies JB, Bruno J, Czeyda-Pommersheim F, et al. Long-term outcome of uterine artery embolization of leiomyomata. *Obstetrics and Gynecology.* Nov 2005;106(5):933–939.
12. Marret H, Cottier JP, Alonso AM, et al. Predictive factors for fibroids recurrence after uterine artery embolisation. *BJOG: An International Journal of Obstetrics and Gynaecology.* Apr 2005;112(4):461–465.
13. Nikolic B, Spies JB, Abbara S, Goodwin SC. Ovarian artery supply of uterine fibroids as a cause of treatment failure after uterine artery embolization: a case report. *Journal of Vascular and Interventional Radiology.* 1999;10(9): 1167–1170.
14. Burn PR, McCall JM, Chinn RJ, et al. Uterine fibroleiomyoma: MR imaging appearances before and after embolization of uterine arteries. *Radiology.* 2000;214(3):729–734.
15. ACOG Committee Opinion. Number 293, February 2004: Uterine Artery Embolization. *Obstetrics and Gynecology.* Feb 2004;103(2):403–404.
16. Ravina JH, Vigneron NC, Aymard A, et al. Pregnancy after embolization of uterine myoma: report of 12 cases. *Fertility and Sterility.* 2000;73(6):1241–1243.

17. McLucas B, Goodwin S, Adler L, et al. Pregnancy following uterine fibroid embolization. *International Journal of Gynaecology and Obstetrics*. 2001;74 (1):1–7.
18. Kovacs P, Stangel JJ, Santoro NF, Lieman H. Successful pregnancy after transient ovarian failure following treatment of symptomatic leiomyomata. *Fertility and Sterility*. 2002;77(6):1292–1295.
19. Pron G, Mocarski E, Bennett J, et al. Pregnancy after uterine artery embolization for leiomyomata: the Ontario multicenter trial. *Obstetrics and Gynecology*. Jan 2005;105(1):67–76.
20. Pelage JP, Le Dref O, Soyer P, et al. Fibroid-related menorrhagia: treatment with superselective embolization of the uterine arteries and midterm followup. *Radiology*. 2000;215(2):428–431.
21. Pron G, Bennett J, Common A, et al. The Ontario Uterine Fibroid Embolization Trial. Part 2. Uterine fibroid reduction and symptom relief after uterine artery embolization for fibroids. *Fertility and Sterility*. Jan 2003;79(1):120–127.
22. Amato P, Roberts A. Transient ovarian failure: a complication of uterine artery embolization. *Fertility and Sterility*. 2000;75(2):438–439.
23. Tulandi T, Sammour A, Valenti D, et al. Ovarian reserve after uterine artery embolization for leiomyomata. *Fertility and Sterility*. 2002;78(1):197–198.
24. Tropeano G, Litwicka K, Di Stasi C, et al. Permanent amenorrhea associated with endometrial atrophy after uterine artery embolization for symptomatic uterine fibroids. *Fertility and Sterility*. Jan 2003;79(1):132–135.
25. Goldberg J, Pereira L, Berghella V. Pregnancy after uterine artery embolization. *Obstetrics and Gynecology*. 2002;100(5):869–872.
26. Vashisht A, Studd J, Carey A, Burn P. Fatal septicaemia after fibroid embolisation. *Lancet*. 1999;354(9175):307–308.
27. Goodwin SC, Bradley LD, Lipman JC, et al. Uterine artery embolization versus myomectomy: a multicenter comparative study. *Fertility and Sterility*. Jan 2006;85(1):14–21.
28. Pinto I, Chimeno P, Romo A, et al. Uterine fibroids: uterine artery embolization versus abdominal hysterectomy for treatment—a prospective, randomized, and controlled clinical trial. *Radiology*. Feb 2003;226(2):425–431.
29. Hehenkamp WJ, Volkers NA, Donderwinkel PF, et al. Uterine artery embolization versus hysterectomy in the treatment of symptomatic uterine fibroids (EMMY trial): peri- and postprocedural results from a randomized controlled trial. *American Journal of Obstetrics and Gynecology*. Nov 2005; 193(5):1618–1629.
30. Mara M, Fucikova Z, Maskova J, et al. Uterine fibroid embolization versus myomectomy in women wishing to preserve fertility: preliminary results of a randomized controlled trial. *European Journal of Obstetrics, Gynecology, and Reproductive Biology*. 2006;126(2):226–233.
31. Gupta J, Sinha A, Lumsden M, Hickey M. Uterine artery embolization for symptomatic uterine fibroids. *Cochrane Database of Systematic Reviews*. 2006(1):CD005073.

32. Edwards RD, Moss JG, Lumsden MA, et al. Uterine-artery embolization versus surgery for symptomatic uterine fibroids. *New England Journal of Medicine.* 2007;356:360–370.

33. Abbara S, Spies JB, Scialli AR, et al. Transcervical expulsion of a fibroid as a result of uterine artery embolization for leiomyomata. *Journal of Vascular and Interventional Radiology.* 1999;10(4):409–411.

34. Berkowitz RP, Hutchins FL, Jr., Worthington-Kirsch RL. Vaginal expulsion of submucosal fibroids after uterine artery embolization. A report of three cases. *Journal of Reproductive Medicine.* 1999;44(4):373–376.

35. Hald K, Langebrekke A, Klow NE, et al. Laparoscopic occlusion of uterine vessels for the treatment of symptomatic fibroids: initial experience and comparison to uterine artery embolization. *American Journal of Obstetrics and Gynecology.* Jan 2004;190(1):37–43.

36. Lichtinger M, Herbert S, Memmolo A. Temporary, transvaginal occlusion of the uterine arteries: a feasibility and safety study. *Journal of Minimally Invasive Gynecology.* Jan–Feb 2005;12(1):40–42.

Chapter 12. Focused Ultrasound Surgery and Other Thermoablative Therapies

1. Grimson WE, Kikinis R, Jolesz FA, Black PM. Image-guided surgery. *Scientific American.* Jun 1999;280(6):62–69.

2. Goldfarb HA. Laparoscopic coagulation of myoma (myolysis). *Obstetrics and Gynecology Clinics of North America.* 1995;22(4):807–819.

3. Goldfarb HA. Bipolar laparoscopic needles for myoma coagulation. *Journal of the American Association of Gynecologic Laparoscopists.* 1995;2(2):175–179.

4. Zreik TG, Rutherford TJ, Palter SF, et al. Cryomyolysis, a new procedure for the conservative treatment of uterine fibroids. *Journal of the American Association of Gynecologic Laparoscopists.* 1998;5(1):33–38.

5. Sewell PE, Arriola RM, Robinette L, Cowan BD. Real-time I-MR-imaging—guided cryoablation of uterine fibroids. *Journal of Vascular and Interventional Radiology.* 2001;12(7):891–893.

6. Cowan BD, Sewell PE, Howard JC, et al. Interventional magnetic resonance imaging cryotherapy of uterine fibroid tumors: preliminary observation. *American Journal of Obstetrics and Gynecology.* 2002;186(6):1183–1187.

7. Law P, Gedroyc WM, Regan L. Magnetic-resonance-guided percutaneous laser ablation of uterine fibroids. *Lancet.* 1999;354(9195):2049–2050.

8. Hindey J, Law P, Hickey M, et al. Clinical outcomes following percutaneous magnetic resonance image guided laser ablation of symptomatic uterine fibroids. *Human Reproduction.* 2002;17(20):2737–2741.

9. Tempany CM, Stewart EA, McDannold N, et al. MR imaging–guided focused ultrasound surgery of uterine leiomyomas: a feasibility study. *Radiology.* Mar 2003;226(3):897–905.

10. Stewart EA, Gedroyc WM, Tempany CM, et al. Focused ultrasound treatment of uterine fibroid tumors: safety and feasibility of a noninvasive thermoablative technique. *American Journal of Obstetrics and Gynecology.* Jul 2003;189(1):48–54.

11. Hindley J, Gedroyc WM, Regan L, et al. MRI guidance of focused ultrasound therapy of uterine fibroids: early results. *American Journal of Roentgenology.* Dec 2004;183(6):1713–1719.

12. Stewart EA. Clinical outcomes of focused ultrasound surgery for the treatment of uterine fibroids. *Fertility and Sterility.* 2006;85(1):22–29.

13. Spies JB, Coyne K, Guaou Guaou N, et al. The UFS-QOL, a new disease-specific symptom and health-related quality of life questionnaire for leiomyomata. *Obstetrics and Gynecology.* 2002;99(2):290–300.

14. Fennessy F, Tempany C, McDannold N, et al. Expanding treatment guidelines leads to increased efficacy and safety for MRI-guided focused ultrasound surgery of uterine leiomyomas. *Radiology.* 2007;24(3):885–893.

15. Leon-Villapalos J, Kaniorou-Larai M, Dziewulski P. Full thickness abdominal burn following magnetic resonance guided focused ultrasound therapy. *Burns.* Dec 2005;31(8):1054–1055.

16. Smart OC, Hindley JT, Regan L, Gedroyc WG. Gonadotropin-releasing hormone and magnetic-resonance-guided ultrasound surgery for uterine leiomyomata. *Obstetrics and Gynecology.* Jul 2006;108(1):49–54.

17. Vaezy S, Fujimoto VY, Walker C, et al. Treatment of uterine fibroid tumors in a nude mouse model using high-intensity focused ultrasound. *American Journal of Obstetrics and Gynecology.* 2000;183(1):6–11.

18. Chan A, Fujimoto V, Moore D, et al. An image-guided high intensity focused ultrasound device for uterine fibroids treatment. *Medical Physics.* 2002;29 (11):2611–2620.

19. Keshavarzi A, Vaezy S, Noble ML, et al. Treatment of uterine fibroid tumors in an in situ rat model using high-intensity focused ultrasound. *Fertility and Sterility.* Sep 2003;80 Suppl 2:761–767.

20. Chan AH, Fujimoto VY, Moore DE, et al. In vivo feasibility of image-guided transvaginal focused ultrasound therapy for the treatment of intracavitary fibroids. *Fertility and Sterility.* Sep 2004;82(3):723–730.

Chapter 13. Hysterectomy

1. Carlson KJ, Miller BA, Fowler FJ, Jr. The Maine Women's Health Study: I. Outcomes of hysterectomy. *Obstetrics and Gynecology.* 1994;83(4):556–565.

2. Kjerulff KH, Rhodes JC, Langenberg PW, Harvey LA. Patient satisfaction with results of hysterectomy. *American Journal of Obstetrics and Gynecology.* Dec 2000;183(6):1440–1447.

3. Kjerulff KH, Langenberg PW, Rhodes JC, et al. Effectiveness of hysterectomy. *Obstetrics and Gynecology.* 2000;95(3):319–326.

4. Farquhar CM, Sadler L, Harvey S, et al. A prospective study of the short-term outcomes of hysterectomy with and without oophorectomy. *Australian and New Zealand Journal of Obstetrics and Gynaecology.* May 2002;42(2): 197–204.

5. Learman LA, Summitt RL, Jr., Varner RE, et al. Hysterectomy versus expanded medical treatment for abnormal uterine bleeding: clinical outcomes in the medicine or surgery trial. *Obstetrics and Gynecology.* May 2004;103(5 Pt 1):824–833.

6. Kuppermann M, Varner RE, Summitt RL, Jr., et al. Effect of hysterectomy vs medical treatment on health-related quality of life and sexual functioning: the medicine or surgery (Ms) randomized trial. *JAMA: Journal of the American Medical Association.* Mar 24 2004;291(12):1447–1455.

7. Andersen TF, Loft A, Bronnum-Hansen H, et al. Complications after hysterectomy. A Danish population based study 1978–1983. *Acta Obstetricia et Gynecologica Scandinavica.* 1993;72(7):570–577.

8. McPherson K, Metcalfe MA, Herbert A, et al. Severe complications of hysterectomy: the VALUE study. *BJOG: An International Journal of Obstetrics and Gynaecology.* Jul 2004;111(7):688–694.

9. Dicker RC, Greenspan JR, Strauss LT, et al. Complications of abdominal and vaginal hysterectomy among women of reproductive age in the United States. The Collaborative Review of Sterilization. *American Journal of Obstetrics and Gynecology.* 1982;144(7):841–848.

10. Hillis SD, Marchbanks PA, Peterson HB. Uterine size and risk of complications among women undergoing abdominal hysterectomy for leiomyomas. *Obstetrics and Gynecology.* 1996;87(4):539–543.

11. Adashi EY. The climacteric ovary as a functional gonadotropin-driven androgen-producing gland. *Fertility and Sterility.* 1994;62(1):20–27.

12. Shifren JL. The role of androgens in female sexual dysfunction. *Mayo Clinic Proceedings.* Apr 2004;79(4 Suppl):S19–24.

13. Buster JE, Kingsberg SA, Aguirre O, et al. Testosterone patch for low sexual desire in surgically menopausal women: a randomized trial. *Obstetrics and Gynecology.* May 2005;105(5 Pt 1):944–952.

14. Nyunt A, Stephen G, Gibbin J, et al. Androgen status in healthy premenopausal women with loss of libido. *Journal of Sex and Marital Therapy.* Jan–Feb 2005;31(1):73–80.

15. Manson JE, Hsia J, Johnson KC, et al. Estrogen plus progestin and the risk of coronary heart disease. *New England Journal of Medicine.* Aug 7 2003;349 (6):523–534.

16. Anderson GL, Limacher M, Assaf AR, et al. Effects of conjugated equine estrogen in postmenopausal women with hysterectomy: the Women's Health Initiative randomized controlled trial. *JAMA: Journal of the American Medical Association.* Apr 14 2004;291(14):1701–1712.

17. Parker WH, Broder MS, Liu Z, et al. Ovarian conservation at the time of hysterectomy for benign disease. *Obstetrics and Gynecology.* Aug 2005;106(2):219–226.

18. Irwin KL, Weiss NS, Lee NC, Peterson HB. Tubal sterilization, hysterectomy, and the subsequent occurrence of epithelial ovarian cancer. *American Journal of Epidemiology.* 1991;134(4):362–369.

19. Hankinson SE, Hunter DJ, Colditz GA, et al. Tubal ligation, hysterectomy, and risk of ovarian cancer. A prospective study. *JAMA: Journal of the American Medical Association* 1993;270(23):2813–2818.

20. Munro MG. Supracervical hysterectomy: . . . a time for reappraisal. *Obstetrics and Gynecology.* Jan 1997;89(1):133–139.

21. Kuppermann M, Summitt RL, Jr., Varner RE, et al. Sexual functioning after total compared with supracervical hysterectomy: a randomized trial. *Obstetrics and Gynecology.* Jun 2005;105(6):1309–1318.

22. Helstrom L, Lundberg PO, Sorbom D, Backstrom T. Sexuality after hysterectomy: a factor analysis of women's sexual lives before and after subtotal hysterectomy. *Obstetrics and Gynecology.* 1993;81(3):357–362.

23. Rhodes JC, Kjerulff KH, Langenberg PW, Guzinski GM. Hysterectomy and sexual functioning. *JAMA: Journal of the American Medical Association.* 1999;282(20):1934–1941.

24. Thakar R, Ayers S, Clarkson P, et al. Outcomes after total versus subtotal abdominal hysterectomy. *New England Journal of Medicine.* 2002;347(17): 1318–1325.

Chapter 14. Traditional Hormonal Therapies

1. Marshall LM, Spiegelman D, Goldman MB, et al. A prospective study of reproductive factors and oral contraceptive use in relation to the risk of uterine leiomyomata. *Fertility and Sterility.* 1998;70(3):432–439.

2. Wise LA, Palmer JR, Harlow BL, et al. Reproductive factors, hormonal contraception, and risk of uterine leiomyomata in African-American women: a prospective study. *American Journal of Epidemiology.* Jan 15 2004;159(2): 113–123.

3. Chiaffarino F, Parazzini F, La Vecchia C, et al. Use of oral contraceptives and uterine fibroids: results from a case-control study. *British Journal of Obstetrics and Gynaecology.* 1999;106(8):857–860.

4. Faerstein E, Szklo M, Rosenshein N. Risk factors for uterine leiomyoma: a practice-based case-control study. I. African-American heritage, reproductive history, body size, and smoking. *American Journal of Epidemiology.* 2001;153 (1):1–10.

5. Stewart EA, Friedman AJ. Steroidal treatment of myomas: preoperative and longterm medical therapy. *Seminars in Reproductive Endocrinology.* 1992;10 (4):344–357.

6. Rein MS, Barbieri RL, Friedman AJ. Progesterone: a critical role in the pathogenesis of uterine myomas. *American Journal of Obstetrics and Gynecology.* 1995;172(1 Pt 1):14–18.

7. Friedman AJ, Barbieri RL, Doubilet PM, et al. A randomized, double-blind trial of a gonadotropin releasing–hormone agonist (leuprolide) with or without medroxyprogesterone acetate in the treatment of leiomyomata uteri. *Fertility and Sterility.* 1988;49(3):404–409.

8. Carr BR, Breslau NA, Peng N, et al. Effect of gonadotropin-releasing hormone agonist and medroxyprogesterone acetate on calcium metabolism: a prospective, randomized, double-blind, placebo-controlled, crossover trial. *Fertility and Sterility.* Nov 2003;80(5):1216–1223.

9. Murphy AA, Kettel LM, Morales AJ, et al. Regression of uterine leiomyomata in response to the antiprogesterone RU 486. *Journal of Clinical Endocrinology and Metabolism.* 1993;76(2):513–517.

10. Eisinger SH, Meldrum S, Fiscella K, et al. Low-dose mifepristone for uterine leiomyomata. *Obstetrics and Gynecology.* 2003;101:243–250.

11. Steinauer J, Pritts EA, Jackson R, Jacoby AF. Systematic review of mifepristone for the treatment of uterine leiomyomata. *Obstetrics and Gynecology.* Jun 2004;103(6):1331–1336.

12. Istre O, Trolle B. Treatment of menorrhagia with the levonorgestrel intrauterine system versus endometrial resection. *Fertility and Sterility.* 2001;76(2): 304–309.

13. Mercorio F, De Simone R, Di Spiezio Sardo A, et al. The effect of a levonorgestrel-releasing intrauterine device in the treatment of myoma-related menorrhagia. *Contraception.* Apr 2003;67(4):277–280.

14. Grigorieva V, Chen-Mok M, Tarasova M, Mikhailov A. Use of a levonorgestrel-releasing intrauterine system to treat bleeding related to uterine leiomyomas. *Fertility and Sterility.* May 2003;79(5):1194–1198.

Chapter 15. GnRH Agonists, Add-Back Therapies, and GnRH Antagonists

1. Filicori M, Hall DA, Loughlin JS, et al. A conservative approach to the management of uterine leiomyoma: pituitary desensitization by a luteinizing hormone-releasing hormone analogue. *American Journal of Obstetrics and Gynecology.* 1983;147(6):726–727.

2. Stewart EA, Friedman AJ. Steroidal treatment of myomas: preoperative and longterm medical therapy. *Seminars in Reproductive Endocrinology.* 1992; 10(4):344–357.

3. Carr BR, Marshburn PB, Weatherall PT, et al. An evaluation of the effect of gonadotropin-releasing hormone analogs and medroxyprogesterone acetate on uterine leiomyomata volume by magnetic resonance imaging: a prospective, randomized, double blind, placebo-controlled, crossover trial. *Journal of Clinical Endocrinology and Metabolism.* 1993;76(5):1217–1223.

4. Friedman AJ, Barbieri RL, Doubilet PM, et al. A randomized, double-blind trial of a gonadotropin releasing–hormone agonist (leuprolide) with or without medroxyprogesterone acetate in the treatment of leiomyomata uteri. *Fertility and Sterility.* 1988;49(3):404–409.

5. Carr BR, Breslau NA, Peng N, et al. Effect of gonadotropin-releasing hormone agonist and medroxyprogesterone acetate on calcium metabolism: a prospective, randomized, double-blind, placebo-controlled, crossover trial. *Fertility and Sterility.* Nov 2003;80(5):1216–1223.

6. Friedman AJ, Daly M, Juneau-Norcross M, et al. Long-term medical therapy for leiomyomata uteri: a prospective, randomized study of leuprolide acetate depot plus either oestrogen-progestin or progestin "add-back" for 2 years. *Human Reproduction.* 1994;9(9):1618–1625.

7. Daniels AM, Daniels JR, Pike MC, Spicer DV. Addition of unopposed low-dose estradiol (E2) to the gonadotropin releasing hormone agonist (GnRHA) deslorelin (D) results in an unexpectedly low incidence of endometrial hyperplasia. *Journal of the Society for Gynecologic Investigation,* Annual Meeting 2003.

8. Walker CL, Burroughs KD, Davis B, et al. Preclinical evidence for therapeutic efficacy of selective estrogen receptor modulators for uterine leiomyoma. *Journal of the Society for Gynecologic Investigation.* 2000;7(4):249–256.

9. Palomba S, Russo T, Orio F, Jr., et al. Effectiveness of combined GnRH analogue plus raloxifene administration in the treatment of uterine leiomyomas: a prospective, randomized, single-blind, placebo-controlled clinical trial. *Human Reproduction.* Dec 2002;17(12):3213–3219.
10. Palomba S, Orio F, Jr, Russo T, et al. Long-term effectiveness and safety of GnRH agonist plus raloxifene administration in women with uterine leiomyomas. *Human Reproduction.* Jun 2004;19(6):1308–1314.
11. Hammar M, Christau S, Nathorst-Boos J, et al. A double-blind, randomised trial comparing the effects of tibolone and continuous combined hormone replacement therapy in postmenopausal women with menopausal symptoms. *British Journal of Obstetrics and Gynaecology.* 1998;105(8):904–911.
12. De Aloysio D, Altieri P, Penacchioni P, et al. Bleeding patterns in recent postmenopausal outpatients with uterine myomas: comparison between two regimens of HRT. *Maturitas.* 1998;29(3):261–264.
13. Somekawa Y, Chiguchi M, Ishiashi T, et al. Efficacy of ipriflavone in preventing adverse effects of leuprolide. *Journal of Clinical Endocrinology and Metabolism.* 2001;86(7):3202–3206.
14. Kettel LM, Murphy AA, Morales AJ, et al. Rapid regression of uterine leiomyomas in response to daily administration of gonadotropin-releasing hormone antagonist. *Fertility and Sterility.* 1993;60(4):642–646.
15. Felberbaum RE, Germer U, Ludwig M, et al. Treatment of uterine fibroids with a slow-release formulation of the gonadotrophin releasing hormone antagonist Cetrorelix. *Human Reproduction.* 1998;13(6):1660–1668.
16. Gonzalez-Barcena D, Alvarez RB, Ochoa EP, et al. Treatment of uterine leiomyomas with luteinizing hormone-releasing hormone antagonist Cetrorelix. *Human Reproduction.* 1997;12(9):2028–2035.

Chapter 16. Innovative Medical Strategies for Treating Uterine Fibroids

1. Murphy AA, Kettel LM, Morales AJ, et al. Regression of uterine leiomyomata in response to the antiprogesterone RU 486. *Journal of Clinical Endocrinology and Metabolism.* 1993;76(2):513–517.
2. Murphy AA, Kettel LM, Morales AJ, et al. Endometrial effects of long-term low-dose administration of RU486. *Fertility and Sterility.* 1995;63(4):761–766.
3. Steinauer J, Pritts EA, Jackson R, Jacoby AF. Systematic review of mifepristone for the treatment of uterine leiomyomata. *Obstetrics and Gynecology.* Jun 2004;103(6):1331–1336.
4. Eisinger SH, Bonfiglio T, Fiscella K, et al. Twelve-month safety and efficacy of low-dose mifepristone for uterine myomas. *Journal of Minimally Invasive Gynecology.* May–Jun 2005;12(3):227–233.
5. Fiscella K, Eisinger SH, Meldrum S, et al. Effect of mifepristone for symptomatic leiomyomata on quality of life and uterine size: a randomized controlled trial. *Obstetrics and Gynecology.* Dec 2006;108(6):1381–1387.
6. Chwalisz K, DeManno D, Garg R, et al. Therapeutic potential for the selective progesterone receptor modulator asoprisnil in the treatment of leiomyomata. *Seminars in Reproductive Medicine.* May 2004;22(2):113–119.

7. Chwalisz K, Perez MC, Demanno D, et al. Selective progesterone receptor modulator development and use in the treatment of leiomyomata and endometriosis. *Endocrine Reviews.* May 2005;26(3):423–438.
8. Walker CL, Burroughs KD, Davis B, et al. Preclinical evidence for therapeutic efficacy of selective estrogen receptor modulators for uterine leiomyoma. *Journal of the Society for Gynecologic Investigation.* 2000;7(4):249–256.
9. Palomba S, Orio F, Morelli M, et al. Raloxifene administration in premenopausal women with uterine leiomyomas: a pilot study. *Journal of Clinical Endocrinology and Metabolism.* 2002;87(8):3603–3608.
10. Palomba S, Russo T, Orio F, Jr., et al. Effectiveness of combined GnRH analogue plus raloxifene administration in the treatment of uterine leiomyomas: a prospective, randomized, single-blind, placebo-controlled clinical trial. *Human Reproduction.* Dec 2002;17(12):3213–3219.
11. Palomba S, Orio F, Jr., Russo T, et al. Long-term effectiveness and safety of GnRH agonist plus raloxifene administration in women with uterine leiomyomas. *Human Reproduction.* Jun 2004;19(6)1308–1314.
12. Marsh EE, Bulun SE. Steroid hormones and leiomyomas. *Obstetrics and Gynecology Clinics of North America.* Mar 2006;33(1):59–67.
13. Minakuchi K, Kawamura N, Tsujimura A, Ogita S. Remarkable and persistent shrinkage of uterine leiomyoma associated with interferon alfa treatment for hepatitis. *Lancet.* 1999;353(9170):2127–2128.
14. De Leo V, la Marca A, Morgante G, et al. Administration of somatostatin analogue reduces uterine and myoma volume in women with uterine leiomyomata. *Fertility and Sterility.* 2001;75(3):632–633.
15. Nowak RA. Novel therapeutic strategies for leiomyomas: targeting growth factors and their receptors. *Environmental Health Perspectives.* 2000;108 Suppl 5:849–853.
16. Nowak RA. Identification of new therapies for leiomyomas: what in vitro studies can tell us. *Clinical Obstetrics and Gynecology.* 2001;44(2):327–334.
17. Lee BS, Margolin SB, Nowak RA. Pirfenidone: a novel pharmacological agent that inhibits leiomyoma cell proliferation and collagen production. *Journal of Clinical Endocrinology and Metabolism.* 1998;83(1):219–223.
18. Houston KD, Copland JA, Broaddus RR, et al. Inhibition of proliferation and estrogen receptor signaling by peroxisome proliferator-activated receptor gamma ligands in uterine leiomyoma. *Cancer Research.* Mar 15 2003;63(6): 1221–1227.
19. Niu H, Simari RD, Zimmermann EM, Christman GM. Nonviral vector-mediated thymidine kinase gene transfer and ganciclovir treatment in leiomyoma cells. *Obstetrics and Gynecology.* 1998;91(5 Pt 1):735–740.

Chapter 17. The Genetics of Fibroids

1. Watson JD, Crick FH. Molecular structure of nucleic acids; a structure for deoxyribose nucleic acid. *Nature.* Apr 25 1953;171(4356):737–738.
2. Watson JD, Crick FH. Genetical implications of the structure of deoxyribonucleic acid. *Nature.* May 30 1953;171(4361):964–967.
3. Treloar SA, Martin NG, Dennerstein L, et al. Pathways to hysterectomy: insights from longitudinal twin research. *American Journal of Obstetrics and Gynecology.* 1992;167(1):82–88.

4. Snieder H, MacGregor AJ, Spector TD. Genes control the cessation of a woman's reproductive life: a twin study of hysterectomy and age at menopause. *Journal of Clinical Endocrinology and Metabolism.* Jun 1998;83 (6):1875–1880.
5. Vikhlyaeva EM, Khodzhaeva ZS, Fantschenko ND. Familial predisposition to uterine leiomyomas. *International Journal of Gynaecology and Obstetrics.* Nov 1995;51(2):127–131.
6. Van Voorhis BJ, Romitti PA, Jones MP. Family history as a risk factor for development of uterine leiomyomas. Results of a pilot study. *Journal of Reproductive Medicine.* Aug 2002;47(8):663–669.
7. Tomlinson IP, Alam NA, Rowan AJ, et al. Germline mutations in FH predispose to dominantly inherited uterine fibroids, skin leiomyomata and papillary renal cell cancer. *Nature Genetics.* 2002;30(4):406–410.
8. Toro JR, Nickerson ML, Wei MH, et al. Mutations in the fumarate hydratase gene cause hereditary leiomyomatosis and renal cell cancer in families in North America. *American Journal of Human Genetics.* Jul 2003;73(1):95–106.
9. Stewart EA, Morton CC. The genetics of uterine leiomyomata: what clinicians need to know. *Obstetrics and Gynecology.* Apr 2006;107(4):917–921.
10. Reed WB, Walker R, Horowitz R. Cutaneous leiomyomata with uterine leiomyomata. *Acta Dermato-Venereologica.* 1973;53(5):409–416.
11. Marsh DJ, Dahia PL, Zheng Z, et al. Germline mutations in PTEN are present in Bannayan-Zonana syndrome. *Nature Genetics.* 1997;16(4):333–334.
12. Rein MS, Friedman AJ, Barbieri RL, et al. Cytogenetic abnormalities in uterine leiomyomata. *Obstetrics and Gynecology.* 1991;77(6):923–926.
13. Brosens I, Deprest J, Dal Cin P, Van den Berghe H. Clinical significance of cytogenetic abnormalities in uterine myomas. *Fertility and Sterility.* 1998;69 (2):232–235.
14. Schoenberg Fejzo M, Ashar HR, Krauter KS, et al. Translocation breakpoints upstream of the HMGIC gene in uterine leiomyomata suggest dysregulation of this gene by a mechanism different from that in lipomas. *Genes, Chromosomes and Cancer.* 1996;17(1):1–6.
15. Zhou X, Benson KF, Ashar HR, Chada K. Mutation responsible for the mouse pygmy phenotype in the developmentally regulated factor HMGI-C. *Nature.* 1995;376(6543):771–774.
16. Alam NA, Rowan AJ, Wortham NC, et al. Genetic and functional analyses of FH mutations in multiple cutaneous and uterine leiomyomatosis, hereditary leiomyomatosis and renal cancer, and fumarate hydratase deficiency. *Human Molecular Genetics.* Jun 1 2003;12(11):1241–1252.
17. Pollard P, Wortham N, Barclay E, et al. Evidence of increased microvessel density and activation of the hypoxia pathway in tumours from the hereditary leiomyomatosis and renal cell cancer syndrome. *Journal of Pathology.* Jan 2005;205(1):41–49.
18. Stewart EA, Nowak RA. New concepts in the treatment of uterine leiomyomas. *Obstetrics and Gynecology.* 1998;92(4 Pt 1):624–627.
19. Kiuru M, Lehtonen R, Arola J, et al. Few FH mutations in sporadic counterparts of tumor types observed in hereditary leiomyomatosis and renal cell cancer families. *Cancer Research.* Aug 15 2002;62(16):4554–4557.

20. Gross KL, Panhuysen CI, Kleinman MS, et al. Involvement of fumarate hydratase in nonsyndromic uterine leiomyomas: genetic linkage analysis and FISH studies. *Genes, Chromosomes and Cancer.* Nov 2004;41(3):183–190.
21. Fujimoto J, Hirose R, Sakaguchi H, Tamaya T. Expression of size-polymorphic androgen receptor gene in uterine leiomyoma according to the number of cytosine, adenine, and guanine repeats in androgen receptor alleles. *Tumour Biology.* Jan–Feb 2000;21(1):33–37.
22. Massart F, Becherini L, Gennari L, et al. Genotype distribution of estrogen receptor–alpha gene polymorphisms in Italian women with surgical uterine leiomyomas. *Fertility and Sterility.* Mar 2001;75(3):567–570.
23. Hsieh YY, Chang CC, Tsai FJ, et al. Estrogen receptor thymine-adenine dinucleotide repeat polymorphism is associated with susceptibility to leiomyoma. *Fertility and Sterility.* Jan 2003;79(1):96–99.
24. Al-Hendy A, Salama SA. Catechol-O-methyltransferase polymorphism is associated with increased uterine leiomyoma risk in different ethnic groups. *Journal of the Society for Gynecologic Investigation.* Feb 2006;13(2):136–144.
25. Tsibris JC, Segars J, Coppola D, et al. Insights from gene arrays on the development and growth regulation of uterine leiomyomata. *Fertility and Sterility.* 2002;78(1):114–121.
26. Wang H, Mahadevappa M, Yamamoto K, et al. Distinctive proliferative phase differences in gene expression in human myometrium and leiomyomata. *Fertility and Sterility.* Aug 2003;80(2):266–276.
27. Quade BJ, Wang TY, Sornberger K, et al. Molecular pathogenesis of uterine smooth muscle tumors from transcriptional profiling. *Genes, Chromosomes and Cancer.* Jun 2004;40(2):97–108.
28. Gross K, Morton C, Stewart E. Finding genes for uterine fibroids. *Obstetrics and Gynecology.* 2000;95(4 Suppl 1):S60.

Chapter 18. Pregnancy, Infertility, and Miscarriage

1. Wilcox AJ, Weinberg CR, O'Connor JF, et al. Incidence of early loss of pregnancy. *New England Journal of Medicine.* Jul 28 1988;319(4):189–194.
2. Pritts EA. Fibroids and infertility: a systematic review of the evidence. *Obstetrical and Gynecological Survey.* Aug 2001;56(8):483–491.
3. Garcia CR, Tureck RW. Submucosal leiomyomas and infertility. *Fertility and Sterility.* 1984;42(1):16–19.
4. Farhi J, Ashkenazi J, Feldberg D, et al. Effect of uterine leiomyomata on the results of in-vitro fertilization treatment. *Human Reproduction.* 1995;10 (10):2576–2578.
5. Eldar-Geva T, Meagher S, Healy DL, et al. Effect of intramural, subserosal, and submucosal uterine fibroids on the outcome of assisted reproductive technology treatment. *Fertility and Sterility.* 1998;70:687–691.
6. Rice JP, Kay HH, Mahony BS. The clinical significance of uterine leiomyomas in pregnancy. *American Journal of Obstetrics and Gynecology.* 1989; 160(5 Pt 1):1212–1216.
7. Coronado GD, Marshall LM, Schwartz SM. Complications in pregnancy, labor, and delivery with uterine leiomyomas: a population-based study. *Obstetrics and Gynecology.* 2000;95(5):764–769.

8. Pron G, Bennett J, Common A, et al. The Ontario Uterine Fibroid Embolization Trial. Part 2. Uterine fibroid reduction and symptom relief after uterine artery embolization for fibroids. *Fertility and Sterility.* Jan 2003;79(1): 120–127.

9. Pron G, Mocarski E, Bennett J, et al. Pregnancy after uterine artery embolization for leiomyomata: the Ontario multicenter trial. *Obstetrics and Gynecology.* Jan 2005;105(1):67–76.

Chapter 19. Adenomyosis and Endometrial Polyps

1. Vercellini P, Parazzini F, Oldani S, et al. Adenomyosis at hysterectomy: a study on frequency distribution and patient characteristics. *Human Reproduction.* 1995;10(5):1160–1162.

2. Raju GC, Naraynsingh V, Woo J, Jankey N. Adenomyosis uteri: a study of 416 cases. *Australian and New Zealand Journal of Obstetrics and Gynecology.* 1988;28(72):72–73.

3. Stewart EA, Strauss JF. Disorders of the uterus: leiomyomas, adenomyosis, endometrial polyps, abnormal uterine bleeding, intrauterine adhesions and dysmenorrhea. In: Barbieri RL, Strauss JF, eds. *Yen and Jaffe's Reproductive Endocrinology.* 5th ed. Philadelphia: Elsevier, 2004:713–734.

4. Mori T, Singtripop T, Kawashima S. Animal model of uterine adenomyosis: is prolactin a potent inducer of adenomyosis in mice? *American Journal of Obstetrics and Gynecology.* 1991;165:232–234.

5. Tamai K, Togashi K, Ito T, et al. MR imaging findings of adenomyosis: correlation with histopathologic features and diagnostic pitfalls. *Radiographics.* Jan–Feb 2005;25(1):21–40.

6. Duehold M, Lundorf E, Hansen ES, et al. Magnetic resonance imaging and transvaginal ultrasonography for the diagnosis of adenomyosis. *Fertility and Sterility.* 2001;76(3):588–594.

7. Igarashi M, Abe Y, Fukuda M, et al. Novel conservative medical therapy for uterine adenomyosis with a danazol-loaded intrauterine device. *Fertility and Sterility.* 2000;74(2):412–413.

8. Lass A, Williams G, Abusheikha N, Brinsden P. The effect of endometrial polyps on outcomes of IVF cycles. *Journal of Assisted Reproduction and Genetics.* 1999;16(8):410–415.

9. Van Bogaert LJ. Clinicopathologic findings in endometrial polyps. *Obstetrics and Gynecology.* 1988;71:771–773.

10. Chavez NF, Garner EO, Khan W, et al. Does the introduction of new technology change population demographics? Minimally invasive technologies and endometrial polyps. *Gynecologic and Obstetric Investigation.* 2002;54(4): 217–220.

11. Clevenger-Hoeft M, Syrop CH, Stovall DW, Van Voorhis BJ. Sonohysterography in premenopausal women with and without abnormal bleeding. *Obstetrics and Gynecology.* 1999;94(4):516–520.

12. DeWaay DJ, Syrop CH, Nygaard IE, et al. Natural history of uterine polyps and leiomyomata. *Obstetrics and Gynecology.* 2002;100(1):3–7.

13. Brill AI. What is the role of hysteroscopy in the management of abnormal uterine bleeding? *Clinical Obstetrics and Gynecology.* 1995;38(2):319–345.

14. Emanuel MH, Wamsteker K, Lammes FB. Is dilatation and curettage obsolete for diagnosing intrauterine disorders in premenopausal patients with persistent abnormal uterine bleeding? *Acta Obstetricia and Gynecologica Scandinavica.* Jan 1997;76(1):65–68.

Chapter 20. Uterine Cancers

1. Davies JL, Rosenshein NB, Antunes CM, Stolley PD. A review of the risk factors for endometrial carcinoma. *Obstetrical and Gynecological Survey.* 1981;36(3):107–116.
2. Feldman S, Cook EF, Harlow BL, Berkowitz RS. Predicting endometrial cancer among older women who present with abnormal vaginal bleeding. *Gynecologic Oncology.* Mar 1995;56(3):376–381.
3. *Surgical Alternatives to Hysterectomy in the Management of Leiomyomas.* Practice Bulletin No. 16: American College of Obstetricians and Gynecologists; 2000.
4. Kawamura N, Ichimura T, Ito F, et al. Transcervical needle biopsy for the differential diagnosis between uterine sarcoma and leiomyoma. *Cancer.* Mar 15 2002;94(6):1713–1720.
5. Leibsohn S, d'Ablaing G, Mishell DR, Jr., Schlaerth JB. Leiomyosarcoma in a series of hysterectomies performed for presumed uterine leiomyomas. *American Journal of Obstetrics and Gynecology.* 1990;162(4):968–974; discussion 974–976.
6. Schwartz LB, Diamond MP, Schwartz PE. Leiomyosarcomas: clinical presentation. *American Journal of Obstetrics and Gynecology.* 1993;168(1 Pt 1): 180–183.
7. Parker WH, Fu YS, Berek JS. Uterine sarcoma in patients operated on for presumed leiomyoma and rapidly growing leiomyoma. *Obstetrics and Gynecology.* 1994;83(3):414–418.
8. Harlow BL, Weiss NS, Lofton S. The epidemiology of sarcomas of the uterus. *Journal of the National Cancer Institute.* 1986;76(3):399–402.
9. Wysowski DK, Honig SF, Beitz J. Uterine sarcoma associated with tamoxifen use. *New England Journal of Medicine.* 2002;346(23):1832–1833.
10. Pattani SJ, Kier R, Deal R, Luchansky E. MRI of uterine leiomyosarcoma. *Magnetic Resonance Imaging.* 1995;13(2):331–333.
11. Tanaka YO, Nishida M, Tsunoda H, et al. Smooth muscle tumors of uncertain malignant potential and leiomyosarcomas of the uterus: MR findings. *Journal of Magnetic Resonance Imaging.* Dec 2004;20(6):998–1007.
12. Loong EP, Wong FW. Uterine leiomyosarcoma diagnosed during treatment with agonist of luteinizing hormone-releasing hormone for presumed uterine fibroid. *Fertility and Sterility.* 1990;54(3):530–531.
13. Meyer WR, Mayer AR, Diamond MP, et al. Unsuspected leiomyosarcoma: treatment with a gonadotropin-releasing hormone analogue. *Obstetrics and Gynecology.* 1990;75(3 Pt 2):529–532.
14. Common AA, Mocarski EJ, Kolin A, et al. Therapeutic failure of uterine fibroid embolization caused by underlying leiomyosarcoma. *Journal of Vascular and Interventional Radiology.* Dec 2001;12(12):1449–1452.

15. Friedman AJ, Haas ST. Should uterine size be an indication for surgical intervention in women with myomas? *American Journal of Obstetrics and Gynecology.* 1993;168(3 Pt 1):751–755.
16. Kawamura N, Ito F, Ichimura T, et al. Transient rapid growth of uterine leiomyoma in a postmenopausal woman. *Oncology Reports.* Nov–Dec 1999; 6(6):1289–1292.

Chapter 21. Fibroid-like Conditions

1. Walker CL, Stewart EA. Uterine fibroids: the elephant in the room. *Science.* June 10 2005;308(5728):1589–1592.
2. Suginami H, Kaura R, Ochi H, Matsuura S. Intravenous leiomyomatosis with cardiac extension: successful surgical management and histopathologic study. *Obstetrics and Gynecology.* Sep 1990;76(3 Pt 2):527–529.
3. Clement PB, Young RH, Scully RE. Intravenous leiomyomatosis of the uterus. A clinicopathological analysis of 16 cases with unusual histologic features. *American Journal of Surgical Pathology.* Dec 1988;12(12):932–945.
4. Uchida H, Hattori Y, Nakada K, Iida T. Successful one-stage radical removal of intravenous leiomyomatosis extending to the right ventricle. *Obstetrics and Gynecology.* May 2004;103(5 Pt 2):1068–1070.
5. Tresukosol D, Kudelka AP, Malpica A, et al. Leuprolide acetate and intravascular leiomyomatosis. *Obstetrics and Gynecology.* Oct 1995;86(4 Pt 2):688–692.
6. Mitsuhashi A, Nagai Y, Sugita M, et al. GnRH agonist for intravenous leiomyomatosis with cardiac extension. A case report. *Journal of Reproductive Medicine.* Oct 1999;44(10):883–886.
7. Dal Cin P, Quade BJ, Neskey DM, et al. Intravenous leiomyomatosis is characterized by a der(14)t(12;14)(q15;q24). *Genes, Chromosomes and Cancer.* Feb 2003;36(2):205–206.
8. Akkersdijk GJ, Flu PK, Giard RW, et al. Malignant leiomyomatosis peritonealis disseminata. *American Journal of Obstetrics and Gynecology.* Aug 1990;163(2):591–593.
9. Butnor KJ, Burchette JL, Robboy SJ. Progesterone receptor activity in leiomyomatosis peritonealis disseminata. *International Journal of Gynecological Pathology.* Jul 1999;18(3):259–264.
10. Danikas D, Goudas VT, Rao CV, Brief DK. Luteinizing hormone receptor expression in leiomyomatosis peritonealis disseminata. *Obstetrics and Gynecology.* Jun 2000;95(6 Pt 2):1009–1011.
11. Parente JT, Levy J, Chinea F, et al. Adjuvant surgical and hormonal treatment of leiomyomatosis peritonealis disseminata. A case report. *Journal of Reproductive Medicine.* Jun 1995;40(6):468–470.
12. Heinig J, Neff A, Cirkel U, Klockenbusch W. Recurrent leiomyomatosis peritonealis disseminata after hysterectomy and bilateral salpingo-oophorectomy during combined hormone replacement therapy. *European Journal of Obstetrics, Gynecology and Reproductive Biology.* Dec 10 2003;111(2):216–218.

13. Quade BJ, McLachlin CM, Soto-Wright V, et al. Disseminated peritoneal leiomyomatosis. Clonality analysis by X chromosome inactivation and cytogenetics of a clinically benign smooth muscle proliferation. *American Journal of Pathology.* Jun 1997;150(6):2153–2166.
14. Fujii S, Nakashima N, Okamura H, et al. Progesterone-induced smooth muscle-like cells in the subperitoneal nodules produced by estrogen. Experimental approach to leiomyomatosis peritonealis disseminata. *American Journal of Obstetrics and Gynecology.* Jan 15 1981;139(2):164–172.
15. Yu J, Astrinidis A, Howard S, Henske EP. Estradiol and tamoxifen stimulate lymphangiomyomatosis-associated angiomyolipoma cell growth and activate both genomic and non-genomic signaling pathways. *American Journal of Physiology. Lung Cellular and Molecular Physiology.* Apr 2004;286(4):L694–700.
16. Smolarek TA, Wessner LL, McCormack FX, et al. Evidence that lymphangiomyomatosis is caused by TSC2 mutations: chromosome 16p13 loss of heterozygosity in angiomyolipomas and lymph nodes from women with lymphangiomyomatosis. *American Journal of Human Genetics.* Apr 1998;62(4):810–815.
17. Carsillo T, Astrinidis A, Henske EP. Mutations in the tuberous sclerosis complex gene TSC2 are a cause of sporadic pulmonary lymphangioleiomyomatosis. *Proceedings of the National Academy of Sciences of the United States of America.* May 23 2000;97(11):6085–6090.
18. Taylor JR, Ryu J, Colby TV, Raffin TA. Lymphangioleiomyomatosis. Clinical course in 32 patients. *New England Journal of Medicine.* Nov 1 1990;323(18):1254–1260.
19. Whale CI, Johnson SR, Phillips KG, et al. Lymphangioleiomyomatosis: a case-control study of perinatal and early life events. *Thorax.* Nov 2003;58(11):979–982.
20. NHLBI Workshop Summary. Report of workshop on lymphangioleiomyomatosis. National Heart, Lung, and Blood Institute. *American Journal of Respiratory and Critical Care Medicine.* Feb 1999;159(2):679–683.
21. Hancock E, Osborne J. Lymphangioleiomyomatosis: a review of the literature. *Respiratory Medicine.* Jan 2002;96(1):1–6.
22. Banner AS, Carrington CB, Emory WB, et al. Efficacy of oophorectomy in lymphangioleiomyomatosis and benign metastasizing leiomyoma. *New England Journal of Medicine.* Jul 23 1981;305(4):204–209.
23. Ho AY, Lam B, Ooi CC, et al. High dose progesterone therapy in lymphangioleiomyomatosis: a case report and review of literature. *Chinese Medical Journal* (Engl). Aug 1998;111(8):759–761.
24. McCarty KS, Jr., Mossler JA, McLelland R, Sieker HO. Pulmonary lymphangiomyomatosis responsive to progesterone. *New England Journal of Medicine.* Dec 18 1980;303(25):1461–1465.
25. Henske EP. Metastasis of benign tumor cells in tuberous sclerosis complex. *Genes, Chromosomes and Cancer.* Dec 2003;38(4):376–381.

26. Karbowniczek M, Astrinidis A, Balsara BR, et al. Recurrent lymphangiomy-omatosis after transplantation: genetic analyses reveal a metastatic mecha-nism. *American Journal of Respiratory and Critical Care Medicine.* Apr 1 2003;167(7):976–982.

27. Hayashi T, Fleming MV, Stetler-Stevenson WG, et al. Immunohistochemical study of matrix metalloproteinases (MMPs) and their tissue inhibitors (TIMPs) in pulmonary lymphangioleiomyomatosis (LAM). *Human Patholo-gy.* Sep 1997;28(9):1071–1078.

28. Cramer SF. Pulmonary lymphangiomyomatosis and metastasizing leiomy-oma. *New England Journal of Medicine.* Sep 3 1981;305(10):587–588.

29. Peters WA, III, Howard DR, Andersen WA, Figge DC. Uterine smooth-muscle tumors of uncertain malignant potential. *Obstetrics and Gynecology.* Jun 1994;83(6):1015–1020.

30. Quade BJ. Pathology, cytogenetics and molecular biology of uterine leiomy-omas and other smooth muscle lesions. *Current Opinion in Obstetrics and Gynecology.* Feb 1995;7(1):35–42.

Appendix. Hints for Surgical Recovery

1. Phillips DM. JCAHO pain management standards are unveiled. Joint Com-mission on Accreditation of Healthcare Organizations. *JAMA: Journal of the American Medical Association.* Jul 26 2000;284(4):428–429.

2. Kaufman E, Epstein JB, Gorsky M, et al. Preemptive analgesia and local anes-thesia as a supplement to general anesthesia: a review. *Anesthesia Progress.* Spring 2005;52(1):29–38.

3. Chavez NF, Zweizig SL, Stewart EA. Neuropathic uterine pain after hys-terectomy. A case report. *Journal of Reproductive Medicine.* Jun 2003;48(6):466–468.

4. Belgrade MJ. Following the clues to neuropathic pain. Distribution and other leads reveal the cause and the treatment approach. *Postgraduate Medicine.* Nov 1999;106(6):127–132, 135–140.

5. Weir LF, Nygaard IE, Wilken J, et al. Postoperative activity restrictions: any evidence? *Obstetrics and Gynecology.* Feb 2006;107(2):305–309.

Index

genetic factors *(continued)*
138–39, 141, 161, 163; in intravenous
leiomyomatosis, 167; molecular genetics, 140–42; tumor suppressor genes,
141; twin studies of, 137–38
Gleevec, 22–23, 137
gonadotropin-releasing hormone
(GnRH), 26, 28*f*, 29, 39, 121
gonadotropin-releasing hormone
(GnRH) agonists, 59, 64, 77, 103,
113, 119, 121–23; add-back therapies
and, 123–25; for adenomyosis, 156;
for anemia, 77–78, 123; formulations
of, 77, 123; for intravenous
leiomyomatosis, 166; limitations of,
122–23; mechanism of action of,
121–22; side effects of, 122
gonadotropin-releasing hormone
(GnRH) antagonists, 125
gonadotrophins, 27, 28*f*
growth factors, 34–36
growth hormone (GH), 34, 129

halofuginone, 129
health care costs, 25
heart disease, 20–22, 107, 165–66
hematologic disorders, 54–55
hereditary leiomyomatosis and renal cell
carcinoma (HLRCC), 138–39, 141,
161, 163
high blood pressure, 20–21
high intensity focused ultrasound, 97
hirsutism, 124
HMGA2 gene, 140–41
home modifications after surgery, 185
hormonal treatment, 117–29; add-back
therapies, 123–24; birth control pills
and progestin, 117–20; GnRH
agonists, 121–23; GnRH antagonists,
125; innovative steroidal therapies,
126–27; nonsteroidal, 128–29
hormone blockers, 30
hormone replacement therapy, 107, 190
hormones, 26–36, 37. *See also*
endocrinology
hot flashes, 78, 122, 126
human papilloma virus (HPV), 108
hydrotherm endometrial ablation, 67*t*

hypothalamus, 26–29, 28*f*
hysterectomy, 19, 24, 30, 104–13; for
adenomyosis, 156; advantages of, 104;
GnRH agonists and, 113; laparoscopic,
112–13; pelvic prolapse after, 109–10;
recovery after, 25, 179–90; with
removal of cervix, 105, 106*f*, 108–12;
with removal of ovaries, 105, 106*f*,
107–8, 162; risks of, 104–5; sexual
function after, 109, 111; surgical
approach for, 112–13; types of,
105–12, 106*f*; for uterine sarcoma,
162, 163–64; vaginal vs. abdominal,
105, 112–13; for women at risk for
uterine cancer, 163–64
hysterosalpingogram (HSG), pl. 3,
46–47, 95
hysteroscopic myomectomy, pl. 6,
63–65; advantages of, 64; endometrial
ablation and, 66; fibroid size for, 64;
fluids for, 65; instruments for, 64–65;
pregnancy after, 146, 150
hysteroscopy, pl. 2, pl. 6, 46;
endometrial polyps on, pl. 2, 158

ibuprofen, 181–82, 183
image-guided therapy, 95
imatinib mesylate, 22–23, 137
incidence of fibroids, 7–8
incisions for abdominal myomectomy,
79–81
infection, postoperative, 81
infertility: endometrial polyps and, 157;
evaluation for, 145; fibroids and,
146–47; after uterine artery
embolization, 89–90
insulin, 34, 36
insulin-like growth factor (IGF), 36, 129
interferon, 128–29
intramural fibroids, 14, 15*f*
intrauterine device (IUD), 33, 34; for
adenomyosis, 156; for endometrial
ablation, 68
intravenous leiomyomatosis (IVL),
165–67; development of, 167;
diagnosis of, 166; genetics of, 167;
treatment of, 166–67
in vitro fertilization (IVF), 125, 146–47

progesterone, 27–29, 28*f*, 30–32, 36, 118; in fibroid formation, 9, 38–39, 118–19; GnRH effects on, 78; leiomyomatosis peritonealis disseminata and, 167–68; during menstrual cycle, 119; receptors for, 33, 128
progesterone receptor modulators (PRMs), 32, 127
progestins, 9, 30–33; add-back therapies, 123–24; in birth control pills, 117–18; for leiomyomatosis peritonealis disseminata, 168; treatment with, 118–19
prolactin, 29, 155
prophylactic myomectomy, 52
prostaglandins, 181
protein hormones, 34, 35*f*
PTEN gene, 141
pulmonary embolus (PE), 81, 99

race: fibroid incidence and, 8, 9, 24, 58; keloids and, 16, 39; uterine artery embolization and, 93; uterine sarcoma and, 162
raloxifene, 124, 127
recurrence of fibroids, 52, 56–59, 70, 75; clinical, 57; genotype and, 137; risk factors for, 57–59; subclinical, 56
Reed's syndrome, 139
renal angiomyolipoma, 168
renal cell carcinoma and fibroids, 138–39, 141, 161, 163
reproductive endocrinology and infertility (REI) specialists, 145
research, 175–76
resectoscope, 64–65, 67*t*
risk factors for fibroids, 8–9
RNA, 134

sagittal scan, 43*f*, 50
saline-infusion sonogram (SIS), pl. 1, 44–46, 45*f*
salpingo-oophorectomy, bilateral, 105, 106*f*, 107–8
sanitary products, 3–4, 25, 173–74
scar tissue, 16, 36
sciatica, 4
second messengers, 34, 35*f*

selective estrogen receptor modulators (SERMs), 30, 31*f*, 32, 124, 127
selective progesterone receptor modulators (SPRMs), 32, 127
serosa, 10, 11*f*, 15*f*
sexual function, 109, 111
size of fibroids, 12–14, 13*f*; for hysteroscopic myomectomy, 64; ovarian imaging and, 162–63
Smads, 36
smoking, 9, 38; heart disease and, 20–21
smooth muscle cells, 12, 16, 21
somatostatin, 129
sonohysterogram, pl. 1, 44–46
steroid hormones, 29–34; in add-back therapies, 123–24; androgens, 32; in birth control pills, 117–18; delivery routes for, 33; dose of, 32; duration of exposure to, 32–33; estrogen, 29–30; in fibroid formation and growth, 38–39, 118–19; innovative therapies, 126–27; leiomyomatosis peritonealis disseminata and, 167–68; during menstrual cycle, 119; in pregnancy, 119; progesterone, 30–32; receptors for, 30, 31*f*, 33; regulation of, 33
stool softeners, 186
submucosal fibroids, pl. 2, pl. 6, 10, 14, 15*f*; prolapsed, 68–69; staging of, 14, 15*f*, 63–64
subserosal fibroids, 14, 15*f*
supracervical hysterectomy (SCH), 105, 106*f*, 108–12
surgical recovery, 25, 179–90; bathroom safety, 185–86; bowel and bladder function, 186–87; driving, 188–89; emotional health, 189; home preparations, 185; movement, 187–88; nausea, 183–84; pain management, 179–83; surgical menopause, 189–90; things to pack for the hospital, 184–85
surgical treatments, 63–113; abdominal myomectomy, 75–82, 76*f*; costs of, 25; endometrial ablation, 65–68, 67*t*; focused ultrasound surgery, 49, 95–103, 98*f*; hysterectomy, 104–13; hysteroscopic myomectomy, pl. 6, 63–65; laparoscopic myomectomy,